VALVE SURGERY AT THE TURN OF THE MILLENNIUM

Developments in Cardiovascular Medicine

232. A. Bayés de Luna, F. Furlanello, B.J. Maron and D.P. Zipes (eds.):
Arrhythmias and Sudden Death in Athletes. 2000 ISBN: 0-7923-6337-X
233. J-C. Tardif and M.G. Bourassa (eds): *Antioxidants and Cardiovascular Disease.*
2000. ISBN: 0-7923-7829-6
234. J. Candell-Riera, J. Castell-Conesa, S. Aguadé Bruiz (eds): *Myocardium at
Risk and Viable Myocardium Evaluation by SPET.* 2000.ISBN: 0-7923-6724-3
235. M.H. Ellestad and E. Amsterdam (eds): Exercise Testing: New Concepts for the
New Century. 2001. ISBN: 0-7923-7378-2
236. Douglas L. Mann (ed.): The Role of Inflammatory Mediators in the Failing
Heart. 2001 ISBN: 0-7923-7381-2
237. Donald M. Bers (ed.): Excitation-Contraction Coupling and Cardiac
Contractile Force, Second Edition. 2001 ISBN: 0-7923-7157-7
238. Brian D. Hoit, Richard A. Walsh (eds.): Cardiovascular Physiology in the
Genetically Engineered Mouse, Second Edition. 2001 ISBN 0-7923-7536-X
239. Pieter A. Doevendans, A.A.M. Wilde (eds.): Cardiovascular Genetics for Clinicians
2001 ISBN 1-4020-0097-9
240. Stephen M. Factor, Maria A.Lamberti-Abadi, Jacobo Abadi (eds.): Handbook of
Pathology and Pathophysiology of Cardiovascular Disease. 2001
ISBN 0-7923-7542-4
241. Liong Bing Liem, Eugene Downar (eds): Progress in Catheter Ablation. 2001
ISBN 1-4020-0147-9
242. Pieter A. Doevendans, Stefan Kääb (eds): Cardiovascular Genomics: New
Pathophysiological Concepts. 2002 ISBN 1-4020-7022-5
243. Daan Kromhout, Alessandro Menotti, Henry Blackburn (eds.): Prevention
of Coronary Heart Disease: Diet, Lifestyle and Risk Factors in the Seven
Countries Study. 2002 ISBN 1-4020-7123-X
244. Antonio Pacifico (ed.), Philip D. Henry, Gust H. Bardy, Martin Borggrefe,
Francis E. Marchlinski, Andrea Natale, Bruce L. Wilkoff (assoc. eds):
Implantable Defibrillator Therapy: A Clinical Guide. 2002 ISBN 1-4020-7143-4
245. Hein J.J. Wellens, Anton P.M. Gorgels, Pieter A. Doevendans (eds.):
The ECG in Acute Myocardial Infarction and Unstable Angina: Diagnosis and Risk
Stratification. 2002 ISBN 1-4020-7214-7
246. Jack Rychik, Gil Wernovsky (eds.): Hypoplastic Left Heart Syndrome. 2003
ISBN 1-4020-7319-4
247. Thomas H. Marwick: Stress Echocardiography. Its Role in the Diagnosis and Evaluation
of Coronary Artery Disease 2nd Edition. ISBN 1-4020-7369-0
248. Akira Matsumori: Cardiomyopathies and Heart Failure: Biomolecular, Infectious
and Immune Mechanisms. 2003 ISBN 1-4020-7438-7
249. Ralph Shabetai: The Pericardium. 2003 ISBN 1-4020-7639-8
250. Irene D. Turpie; George A. Heckman (eds.): Aging Issues in Cardiology. 2004
ISBN 1-40207674-6
251. C.H. Peels; L.H.B. Baur (eds.): Valve Surgery at the Turn of the Millennium. 2004
ISBN 1-4020-7834-X
252. Jason X.-J. Yuan (ed.): Hypoxic Pulmonary Vasoconstriction: Cellular and Molecular
Mechanisms. 2004 ISBN 1-4020-7857-9

Previous volumes are still available

VALVE SURGERY AT THE TURN OF THE MILLENNIUM

edited by

C. H. Peels

*Catharina Hospital
Eindhoven, The Netherlands*

and

L.H.B. Baur

*Atrium Medical Center
Heerlen, The Netherlands*

SPRINGER SCIENCE+BUSINESS MEDIA, LLC

Library of Congress Cataloging-in-Publication Data

Valve surgery at the turn of the millennium / edited by C.H. Peels and L.H.B. Baur.
    p. ; cm. – (Developments in cardiovascular medicine ; 251)
    Includes bibliographical references and index.
    ISBN 978-1-4757-8847-1   ISBN 978-1-4020-7848-4 (eBook)
    DOI 10.1007/978-1-4020-7848-4

    1. Heart valves—Surgery. 2. Heart valves—Diseases—Surgery. I. Peels, C. H. II. Baur, L. H. B. III. Developments in cardiovascular medicine ; v. 251.
    [DNLM: 1. Heart Valve Diseases—surgery. 2. Heart Valve Prosthesis Implantation. WG 169 V215 2004]
RD598.V325 2004
617.4'dc22   2004044076

The Publisher offers discounts on this book for course use and bulk purchases. For further information, send email to <melissa.ramondetta@wkap.com>.

TABLE OF CONTENTS

PAGE 1   PREFACE TO *"VALVE SURGERY AT THE TURN OF THE MILLENNIUM"*
Preface By C.H. Peels and L.H.B. Baur

SECTION I: PRE AND PERIOPERATIVE EVALUATION OF MITRAL VALVE DISEASE

PAGE 3   *CHAPTER 1: PREOPERATIVE EVALUATION OF MITRAL VALVE STENOSIS: WHAT DO WE NEED?*
Dr. L.H.B. Baur

- Assessment of mitral valve stenosis
- Pre-operative Assessment for Surgical Intervention
- Guideline for Treatment of Mitral Valve Stenosis

PAGE 15   *CHAPTER 2: PREOPERATIVE EVALUATION OF MITRAL REGURGITATION: THE CHALLENGE OF OPTIMAL TIMING*
C.H. Peels

- Introduction
- Evaluation of the cause of MR
- Evaluation of the severity of MR
- Left ventricular function and mitral regurgitation
- Why optimal timing
- Factors influencing timing of surgery

PAGE 25   *CHAPTER 3: PERIOPERATIVE TRANSESOPHAGEAL ECHOCARDIOGRAPHY IN MITRAL VALVE SURGERY*
Dr. R.B.A. van den Brink, Prof.dr. B.A.J.M. de Mol

- Introduction
- How to image the mechanism of mitral valve regurgitation by multiplane TEE?
- Anatomy of the valve: The surgeons view
- Anatomy of the valve: The echocardiographers view

- Function of the mitral valve
- Mechanism of mitral regurgitation
- How to assess severity of mitral regurgitation?
- Does intraoperative TEE during mitral valve repair predict early and late mitral valve dysfunction?
- Evaluation of mitral prostheses by transesophagea ehocardiography
- Conclusion

SECTION II: MITRAL VALVE SURGERY: TECHNIQUES

PAGE 45   *CHAPTER 1: LONG-TERM RESULTS OF PROSTHETIC DEVICES IN MITRAL POSITION*
Dr. G.L. van Rijk-Zwikker, Dr. B.J. M. Delemarre,
Prof. dr. R.A.E. Dion

- The Natural History of Mitral Incompetence
- Role of atrial fibrillation
- Pre-operative determinants for late survival
- Postoperative determinants for late survival after mitral valve replacement
- Post-operative thrombo-embolic events and bleeding
- Re-operations
- Endocarditis
- Post-operative pulmonary hypertension
- Structural failure
- Paravalvular Defects
- Valve Thrombosis
- Pannus
- Summary

PAGE 59   *CHAPTER 2: POSTOPERATIVE EVALUATION AFTER MITRAL VALVE SURGERY*
Dr. F. Flachskampf

- Introduction
- General considerations: indications for and goals of the postoperative echo study
- Postoperative evaluation of mitral valve repair
- Postoperative evaluation of mitral valve replacement
- Other typical postoperative problems
- Does the postoperative echo make a difference

SECTION III: PRE AND PERI-OPERATIVE EVALUATION OF AORTIC VALVE DISEASE

PAGE 69   *CHAPTER 1: PREOPERATIVE EVALUATION OF AORTIC INSUFFICIENCY: OPTIMAL TIMING*
C.H. Peels

- Introduction
- Etiology of aortic regurgitation
- Assessment of severity of aortic regurgitation
- Noninvasive follow up in chronic aortic regurgitation
- Timing of surgical intervention
- Factors influencing outcome after surgery for aortic regurgitation
- Summary

PAGE 77   *CHAPTER 2: HEMODYNAMIC EVALUATION OF AORTIC STENOSIS*
Dr. J.M. van Dantzig

- Introduction
- Echocardiographic evaluation of aortic stenosis: Assessment of valve morphology
- Echocardiographic evaluation of aortic stenosis: Assessment of stenosis severity
- Assessment of stenosis severity in low-flow states
- Conclusion

PAGE 85   *CHAPTER 3: THE ROLE OF TRANSESOPHAGEAL ECHOCARDIOGRAPHY IN THE PERI-OPERATIVE PERIOD*
Dr. L.H.B. Baur

- Aortic Valve Disease
- Mitral Valve Disease
- Detection of Ischemia
- Measurement of Systolic Function and Preload

PAGE 93   *CHAPTER 4: EVALUATION OF VALVE DISEASE WITH*
                      NOVEL IMAGING TECHNIQUES
                      Prof. dr. E.E. van der Wall

                      - Technical Aspects in MR Imaging
                      - Contraindications to MR Imaging
                      - Aortic Valve Stenosis
                      - Aortic Valve Insufficiency
                      - Mitral Valve Stenosis
                      - Mitral Valve Regurgitation
                      - Tricuspid Valve Disease
                      - Pulmonic Valve Disease
                      - Mixed Valvular Disease
                      - Prosthetic Valves
                      - Conclusions

SECTION IV: AORTIC VALVE SURGERY: TECHNIQUES AND CHOICE OF PROSTHESES

PAGE 105   *CHAPTER 1: THE PLACE OF TISSUE VALVES IN AORTIC*
                      VALVE SURGERY
                      Prof. dr. H.A. Huysmans

                      -     Introduction
                      -     Porcine xenografts
                      -     Autografts
                      -     Experience and use of tissue valves
                      -     Indications fr the use of tissue valves

PAGE 111   *CHAPTER 2: THE PLACE OF THE ROSS PROCEDURE IN*
                      AORTIC VALVE DISEASE
                      Prof. dr. M. Hazekamp, P. Schoof

                      - Introduction
                      - Technical aspects
                      - Advantages
                      - Disadvantages
                      - Results
                      - Comment

PAGE 117   *CHAPTER 3: IS A MECHANICAL PROSTHESIS ALWAYS*
            THE BEST SOLUTION FOR AN AORTIC VALVE
            REPLACEMENT IN ADULTS?
            A.H.M. van Straten

            - Introduction
            - Hemodynamic performance
            - Valve related morbidity
            - Valve related death
            - Availability
            - Implantation technique
            - Comfort for the patient
            - Discussion

PAGE 125   *CHAPTER 4: POSTOPERATIVE REGRESSION OF LEFT*
            VENTRICULAR HYPERTROPHY
            Dr. L.H.B. Baur, C. H. Peels, J. Kooiker,
            Prof. dr. H.A. Huysmans

            - Introduction
            - Aortic Stenosis
            - Aortic Insufficiency
            - Our own experience in patients with aortic valve disease
            - Influence of etiology on left ventricular remodeling
            - Influence of concomitant coronary artery disease on left
              ventricular remodeling
            - Mitral Insufficiency

PAGE 137   *CHAPTER 5: VALVE PROSTHESIS – PATIENT MISMATCH*
            HOW TO ASSESS IT AND IS IT REALLY A CLINICAL
            PROBLEM?
            Dr. R.B.A. van den Brink, A.P. Yazdanbakhsh,
            Prof. dr. B.A.J.M. de Mol

            - Introduction
            - Assessment of Valve prosthesis – Patient Mismatch (VP- PM)
            - Clinical impact of valve prosthesis – Patient Mismatch
            - Clinical impact of mitral valve prosthesis – Patient Mismatch(MVP-PM)
            - Conclusion

SECTION V: PROBLEMS IN VALVE DISEASE

PAGE 155   *CHAPTER 1: VALVULAR HEART DISEASE:*
IS IT EVER TOO LATE TO OPERATE?
C.H. Peels

- Introduction
- Cardiac arguments: Severe Aortic Stenosis, when not to
  operate?
- Cardiac arguments: Aortic regurgitation, ever too late to operate?
- Cardiac arguments: Mitral regurgitation, when is the operative
  risk prohibitive?
- Cardiac arguments: Mitral stenosis, never too late to operate
- Non-cardiac arguments: Comorbidity influencing the decision to
  defer from operation

PAGE 163   *CHAPTER 2: PROSTHETIC VALVE DYSFUNCTION*
Dr. B.J.M. Delemarre, Dr. G.L. van Rijk-Zwikker,
Prof. dr. R.A.E. Dion

- Introduction
- Prosthesis related dysfunction, orientation
- Prosthesis related dysfunction, subvalvular apparatus
- Dysfunction of the valve prosthesis, structural
- Dysfunction of the valve prosthesis, non structural

PAGE 179   *CHAPTER 3: VALVULAR PATHOLOGY IN PREGNANCY*
Dr. K. Konings, Dr. F.J.M.E. Roumen, Dr. L.H.B. Baur

- Introduction
- Pregnancy and Valve Pathology; Physiological Adaptation
- Stenotic Valve Lesions
- Regurgitant Valve Pathology
- Prosthetic Heart Valves
- Discussion and Conclusions

PAGE 191   *CHAPTER 4: SURGICAL APPROACH OF ACUTE*
            ENDOCARDITIS
            A.H.M. van Straten

            - Introduction
            - Indications for surgical intervention
            - Surgical technique
            - Results of surgery
            - Discussion

PAGE 199   INDEX

List of contributors:

- Dr. L.H.B. Baur, Department of Cardiology, Atrium Medical Center, P.O. 4446, 6401 CX Heerlen, The Netherlands

- Dr. R.B.A. van den Brink, Department of Cardiology, Academical Medical Center, Meibergdreef 9, 1105 AZ Amsterdam, The Netherlands

- Dr. J.M. van Dantzig, Department of Cardiology, Catharina Hospital P.O. 1350, 5602 ZA Eindhoven, The Netherlands

- Dr. B.J.M. Delemarre, Department of Cardiology, Leyenburg Hospital, P.O. 40551, 2504 LN The Hague, The Netherlands

- Dr. F.A. Flachskampf, Department of Cardiology, University of Erlangen, Östliche Stadtmauerstr. 29, 91054 Erlangen, Germany

- Prof. dr. M. Hazekamp, Department of Cardiothoracic Surgery, Leiden University Medical Center, P.O. 9600, 2300 RC Leiden, The Netherlands

- Prof. dr. H.A. Huysmans, Leiden University Medical Center, P.O. 9600, 2300 RC Leiden, The Netherlands

- J. Kooiker, Department of Gynaecology, Atrium Medical Center, P.O. 4446, 6401 CX Heerlen, The Netherlands

- Prof. dr. B.A.J.M. de Mol, Department of Cardiothoracic Surgery, Academical Medical Center, Meibergdreef 9, 1105 AZ Amsterdam, The Netherlands

- C.H. Peels, Department of Cardiology, Catharina Hospital, Eindhoven, P.O. Box 1350, 5602 ZA The Netherlands

- Dr. F.J.M.E. Roumen, Department of Obstetry and Gynaecology, Atrium Medical Center, P.O. 4446, 6401 CX Heerlen, The Netherlands

- Dr. G.L. van Rijk-Zwikker, Department of Cardiothoracic Surgery, Leiden University Medical Center, P.O. 9600, 2300 RC Leiden, The Netherlands

- A.H.M. van Straten, Department of Cardiothoracic Surgery, Catharina Hospital, P.O. 1350, 5602 ZA Eindhoven, The Netherlands

- A.P. Yazdanbakhsk, Department of Cardiology, Academical Medical Center, Meibergdreef 9, 1105 AZ Amsterdam, The Netherlands

- Prof. dr. E.E. van der Wall, Department of Cardiology, Leiden University Medical Center, P.O. 9600, 2300 RC Leiden, The Netherlands

PREFACE TO "VALVE SURGERY AT THE TURN OF THE MILLENNIUM"

Valvular heart disease remains a major cause of morbidity and mortality and is the third most common problem in cardiology and the second in cardiac surgery. About 10% of cardiac surgical cases deal with valve disease and a far greater number of patients are followed closely of which some are treated medically. In the field of management of valvular heart disease exciting advances have been made.

Was invasive evaluation the cornerstone in the examination and diagnosing of patients in previous decades, in the past 10 to 15 years non-invasive methods for diagnosis of the disease and evaluation of disease severity have been developed and validated. Echocardiography is widespread used for this purpose and has greatly improved assessment of valvular lesions, its severity and the consequences of the valvular dysfunction. Echocardiography has in the last decades, not only greatly improved our knowledge of valvular heart disease but also replaced the invasive pre-operative evaluation of almost all valvular disease problems in adult cardiology. Furthermore it allows us to study these patients serially and thus give insight in the natural history of valvular heart disease. Finally, with these non-invasive studies after medical or surgical intervention, precise assessment of changes in valvular and ventricular function is possible and this improves our understanding of the impact of these interventions, an issue especially important in timing surgery properly. In this respect, several functional indices have been developed and tested.

Cooperation of cardiologists and cardiac surgeons in patients with valvular heart disease is essential for optimal care, especially in the important course of surgical intervention. First and for all, optimal timing is of the utmost importance for the patients prognosis after surgery. Furthermore, the procedure of choice has significant impact on the patients daily life and future, in case re-intervention is to be expected. Selection of patients who are beyond repair, is one of the most difficult decisions to make for both professions and is an item to be discussed thoroughly. In these often very ill patients, the option of cardiac surgery as the resolvance of the clinical problem is of course only applicable when it is a realistic one in which prognosis with surgery will improve significantly.

Prosthetic valve function and dysfunction is an issue which is studied by both cardiologists and cardiac surgeons and knowledge in this field is growing. Investigation and discussion on one hand whether a specific valve is suitable for the specific patient and on the other hand about the surgical technique of insertion, should be encouraged and will improve not only our understanding about prosthetic valve function but more importantly improve valve performance in that specific patient.

2

This book contains an overview of the presentations and discussions which took place at the first European Teaching Program of the European Society of Cardiology in September 2000 in Nice, France, concerning valvular heart disease in adult patients considered for valvular surgery. The different chapters deal with native valve disease encountered mostly in the adult patient, the aortic and mitral valve. Special attention is given to the important issue of optimal timing, to the role of echocardiography in the peri-operative period and to assessment of adequate prosthetic valve function and of prosthetic valve dysfunction. New developments in valvular surgery especially of the aortic valve are discussed and the surgical view on choice of valve replacement device and of the approach of endocarditis is highlighted.

The approach of valvular heart disease has changed in the last decades and is still evolving, a dynamic process which should be followed closely by all professionals dealing with these patients in daily practice. This book offers an overview of most issues in this field anno 2000 which we hope will reach all physicians interested and fascinated by valvular heart disease.

Kathinka H. Peels
Leo H. Baur

PREOPERATIVE EVALUATION OF MITRAL VALVE STENOSIS: WHAT DO WE NEED?

Dr. L.H.B. BAUR

Mitral valve stenosis is a disease, causing left ventricular inflow obstruction due to structural abnormalities of the valve. Rheumatic fever is the predominant cause of mitral valve stenosis and a history of rheumatic fever is present in more than 60% of patients with this diasese[1]. Congenital malformation of the mitral valve is rare and mostly seen in children[2]. The pathologic process in rheumatic fever causes leaflet thickening, calcification and chordal fusion. This results in a funnel-shaped mitral apparatus, in which the mitral orifice is decreased in size. Normally, the mitral valve opens to an area of 4 to 6 cm^2. If the mitral valve opening decreases to less than 2.0 to 2.5 cm^2 patients become symptomatic[3]. Overall 10 year survival of asymptomatic untreated patients with mitral stenosis is good with a survival of 80%[4]. However, with the development of symptoms, 10 year survival decreases to only 15%[4,5]. Also the development of atrial fibrillation is associated with a poor prognosis, with a 10 year survival of 25%[4]. Once there is severe pulmonary hypertension, mean survival drops to <3 years[6].

ASSESSMENT OF MITRAL VALVE STENOSIS

History
If patients with mitral stenosis become symptomatic, dyspnea is the main complaint. Symptoms may be exacerbated by any condition, that increases blood flow across the stenotic valve, such as emotional or physical stress, infection, fever, pregnancy or atrial fibrillation with rapid ventricular response. Atrial arrhythmias may develop in up to 40% of patients and may cause sudden intense dyspnea[7]. Hemoptysis is rare and is mostly associated with end-stage mitral stenosis. Chest pain occurs infrequently and has to be differentiated from angina pectoris[8] The pain is due to right ventricular hypertrophy and rarely from atherosclerotic vascular disease[9]. In some patients systemic embolisation is the first symptoms of the disease[7], the risk related to age and the presence of atrial fibrillation.

4

Physical examination
The auscultatory findings in a patient with mitral stenosis are an openingssnap and a diastolic murmur[7]. The first heart sound is accentuated because the prolonged mitral inflow prevents the leaflets from returning to a normal resting position before left ventricular pressure rises at the onset of systole. The rapid rate of pressure rise of the left ventricle then causes the mitral valve to close abruptly. The first heart sound becomes diminished in intensity if the mitral valve is immobile and heavily calcified.

Electrocardiogram
A widened p-wave in the limb leads or a negative P wave in V_1 is a sign of left atrial enlargement. Atrial flutter or atrial fibrillation can be observed frequently.

Chest x-ray
The classical chest X-Ray shows an enlarged left atrium (fig 1 arrows), with a normal left ventricular contour, pulmonary artery enlargement and varying degrees of pulmonary congestion.

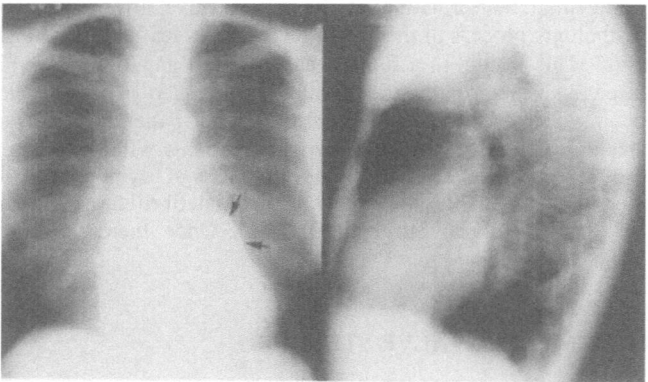

Figure 1: *The classical chest X-Ray shows an enlarged left atrium (arrows), with a normal left ventricular contour, pulmonary artery enlargement and varying degrees of pulmonary congestion.*

Diagnostic testing
Assessment of mitral valve stenosis has changed during the last decades from invasive techniques to non-invasive evaluation with echocardiography and Doppler imaging[10,11]. The role of the catheterization laboratory has changed from a diagnostic tool to a therapeutic tool with the development of percutaneous mitral balloon valvulotomy[12].

Echocardiography
Two dimensional echocardiography is able to identify restricted diastolic opening of the mitral valve leaflets due to "doming" of the anterior leaflet and immobility of the posterior leaflet (fig 2).

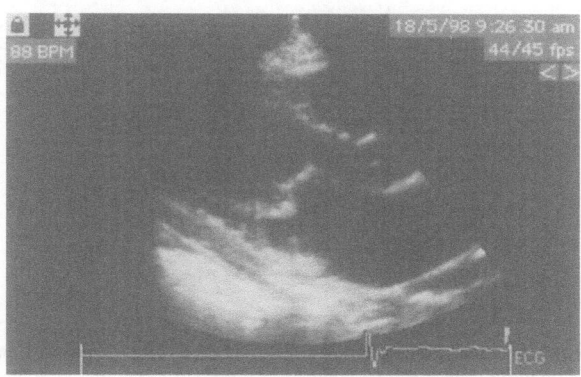

Figure 2: *Parasternal long axis view of a patient with severe mitral stenosis. Typical is diastolic doming of the mitral valve and the hockey-stick appearance of the anterior leaflet.*

Planimetry of the orifice area may be possible from the short-axis view (fig 3)[13]. 2-D echocardiography can also be used to assess the morphological appearance of the mitral valve apparatus, including leaflet mobility, leaflet thickness, leaflet calcification, subvalvular fusion, and the appearance of commissures.
Doppler echocardiography can be used to assess the hemodynamic severity of the obstruction by measurement of the continuous wave Doppler signal across the mitral valve with the modified Bernoulli equation ($\Delta P = 4v^2$)[11]. The transmitral gradient is highly dependent on the RR interval, especially if the patient has atrial fibrillation[14].
Therefore, the average of 6 to 10 beats has to be taken if the patient has atrial fibrillation. The mitral valve area can be non-invasively derived from Doppler echocardiography with either the diastolic half-time method[15] or the continuity equation[16]. Measurement of the diastolic pressure half-time can be obtained from Doppler echocardiography using the deceleration time. The deceleration time is measured by extrapolating the deceleration of early diastolic flow to the baseline and measuring the time from peak mitral inflow velocity to the point of intersection of the deceleration of flow at the baseline. The product of the deceleration time multiplied by 0.29 provides a diastolic pressure half-time. An empiric constant of 220 for derivation of a mitral valve area from the diastolic pressure half-time was proposed by Hatle[11]. The formula for calculating mitral valve area is than: MVA = $220/T_{1/2}$ (MVA is the mitral valve area in cm^2, $T_{1/2}$ is the pressure half-time in ms). This Doppler derived valve area has a good correlation with valve area obtained by cardiac catheterisation and is now universally applied in almost all echocardiographic laboratories. The pressure half-time method may be inaccurate in patients with abnormalities of left

6

atrial or LV compliance, those with associated aortic regurgitation, and those who have had mitral valvulotomy[17].

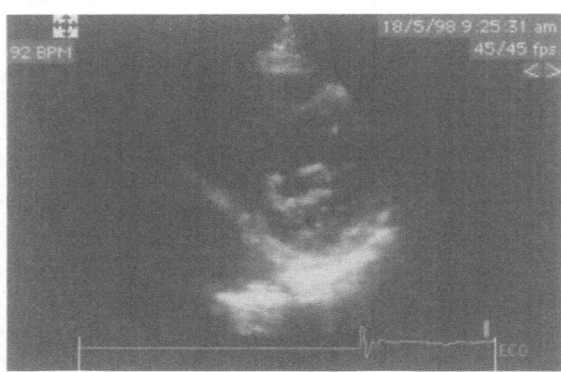

Figure 3: Parasternal short axis view of the same patient (diastolic image). The mitral valve area can easily be traced to calculate area.

The continuity equation is based on the concept that flow remains constant through all heart valves in the absence of valve regurgitation or shunts[18]. Therefore mitral valve area can be calculated by equating flow through the left ventricular outflow tract with flow through the stenotic mitral valve orifice. Volumetric flow through an orifice can be measured by Doppler echocardiography as the product of the valve orifice area and time velocity integral of the Doppler flow through the valve. This gives the following calculation for mitral valve area: $MVA = (LVOT_{area} \times LVOT_{TVI}) / MV_{TVI}$. (MVA is mitral valve area, $LVOT_{area}$ is left ventricular outflow area, $LVOT_{TVI}$ is time velocity integral of left ventricular outflow tract velocity and MV_{TVI} is time velocity integral of the transmitral velocity profile.

In the a-symptomatic patient who has documented mild mitral stenosis (valve area >1.5 cm^2 and mean gradient <5 mm Hg), no further evaluation is needed. These patients usually remain stable for years. If there is more significant mitral stenosis, a decision to proceed further should be based on the suitability of the patient for mitral valvulotomy.

Doppler imaging can also be used to estimate pulmonary artery systolic pressure from the velocity signal of tricuspid regurgitation[19]. Measurement of the right ventricular to right atrial systolic pressure difference can be obtained from the continuous Doppler interrogation of tricuspid regurgitation , applying the modified Bernoulli equation By adding an assumed right atrial pressure, a noninvasive estimation of the pulmonary artery systolic pressure can be obtained.

In patients who lead a sedentary lifestyle, a hemodynamic exercise test with Doppler echocardiography is useful[20]. Objective limitation of exercise tolerance with a rise in transmitral gradient >15 mm Hg and in pulmonary artery systolic pressure >60mmHg may be an indication for percutaneous valvulotomy if the mitral valve morphology is suitable. A small subset of patients has significant limiting symptoms and yet resting hemodynamics that do not indicate moderate to severe mitral stenosis. If there is a discrepancy between symptoms and hemodynamic data, formal exercise testing or dobutamine stress may be useful to differentiate symptoms due to mitral stenosis from other causes of symptoms.

Exercise tolerance, heart rate and blood pressure response, transmitral gradient, and pulmonary artery pressure can be obtained at rest and during exercise. This can usually be accomplished with either supine bicycle or upright exercise with Doppler recording of tricuspid regurgitation and transmitral velocities[21]. Patients who are symptomatic with a significant elevation of pulmonary artery pressure (>60 mm Hg), mean transmitral gradient (>15 mm Hg), or pulmonary artery wedge pressure (≥25 mm Hg) on exertion have hemodynamically significant mitral stenosis and should be considered for further intervention. Alternatively, patients who do not manifest elevation in either pulmonary artery, pulmonary artery wedge, or transmitral pressures coincident with development of symptoms during exercise most likely would not benefit from intervention on the mitral valve.

Echo-Doppler imaging can also be used to assess severity of concomitant aortic valve disease and tricuspid valve disease in patients with mitral valve stenosis.

Cardiac catheterization

Invasive measurement of transmitral gradient and right ventricular pressures is only needed in those patients, in whom further information is required after two-dimensional echocardiographic and Doppler assessment. In all other patients, invasive measurements is redundant and may confuse the doctor if discrepancies are present with non-invasive testing. Most laboratories use the indirect method of measuring left atrial pressure from the pulmonary artery wedge pressure[22].

The accepted approach is measurement of the wedge pressure with a large-bore end hole catheter, firmly wedged into a distal pulmonary artery with a saturation greater than 95%. Pressure measurement is less reliable if a balloon-tipped catheter is used. A dampened pulmonary artery pressure waveform may simulate a true pulmonary artery wedge pressure and may cause a significant overestimation of the transmitral gradient[33]. Even with a properly performed pulmonary wedge pressure, a 40% to 70% overestimation of the transmitral gradient may occur due to delay in the transmission of pressure[33]. The Doppler measurements are consistently more accurate than the gradient obtained by catheterisation[23].

Assessing suitability for valvulotomy

Percutaneous balloon dilatation of the mitral valve is competitive to mitral valve surgery for the treatment of mitral valve stenosis[24,25]. Because not all patients are suitable for percutaneous balloon valvulotomy, patient selection is an important component of successful outcome. Although patient factors (age, NYHA classification and pulmonary artery pressure[26,27]) are important factors determining outcome, mitral valve morphology is the most important factor determining success of mitral valve valvulotomy[28]. Wilkins et al[28] designed a scoring system for patients eligible for mitral valve annuloplasty on the basis of valve characteristics (table 1).

Table 1. Echocardiographic score of the mitral valve

Grade	Mobility	Sub-valvular thickening	Thickening	Calcification
1	Highly mobile valve with only leaflet tips restricted	Minimal thickening just below the mitral leaflets	Leaflets normal in thickness	A single area of increased echo brightness
2	Leaflet mid and base portions have normal mobility	Thickening of chordal structures extending up to one third of the chordal length	Mid-leaflets normal, con-siderable marginal thickening	Scattered areas of brightness confined to leaflet margins
3	Valve continues to move forward in diastole, mainly from the base	Thickening extending to the distal third of the chords	Thickening extending through the entire leaflet	Brightness extending into the mid-portion of the leaflets
4	No or minimal forward movement of leaflets in diastole	Extensive thickening and shortening of all chordal structures extending down to the papillary muscles	Considerable thickening of all leaflet tissue	Extensive brightness throughout much of the leaflet tissue

The total echocardiographic score is derived from an analysis of mitral leaflet mobility, valvular and sub-valvular thickening, and calcification which is graded from 0-4 according to the above criteria. This gives a total score of 0 to 16. As indicated in table 2, patients with a mitral valve score < 8 have a event free survival of more than 90% at 4 years, whereas patients with a score > 8 have a event free survival of less than 40%.

Table 2: Echocardiographic Prediction of outcome of mitral valve balloon angioplasty[29]

Study (reference)	Mean follow-up (months)	Echo criteria	Survival	Survival free of events
Cohen [26]	36 ± 20	Score ≤ 8		68 % at 5 y
		Score ≥ 8		28 % at 5 y
Palacios[30]	20 ± 12	Score ≤ 8	98 % at 4 y	98% at 4 y
		Score ≥ 8	72 % at 4 y	39% at 4 y
Dean [31]	38 ± 16	Score < 8	95 % at 4 y	
		Score 8-12	83 % at 4 y	
		Score > 12	24 % at 4 y	
Cannan [22]	22 ± 10	Com Ca -		86% at 3 y
		Com Ca +	.	40% at 3 y

If a patient is eligible for balloon valvulotomy, a transesophageal echocardiogram has to be performed to exclude left atrial thrombus and quantify any mitral regurgitation[33]. Patients with a thrombus in the left atrial appendage should not undergo percutaneous mitral balloon valvulotomy until the thrombus has been resolved with appropriate anticoagulation. If mitral regurgitation more than grade 3 is present before valvulotomy, the procedure should not be performed.

PRE-OPERATIVE ASSESSMENT FOR SURGICAL INTERVENTION

Surgical treatment of mitral valve stenosis can be a closed commisurotomy, open commisurotomy or mitral valve replacement. Closed commisurotomy, which was very popular in the beginning of the 20th century is now replaced by open commisurotomy and mitral valve replacement. The success of surgical commisurotomy depends on the underlying morphology of the mitral valve apparatus. Optimal results can be achieved in patients with a pliable, non-calcified valve with minimal fusion of the sub-valvular apparatus. Transthoracic and transesophageal echocardiography can determine the suitability of the patient for surgical commisurotomy and may guide the surgeon in the assessment of valvuloplasty[34]. Those patients with heavily calcified valves and more than grade 2 mitral insufficiency have to undergo mitral valve replacement.

GUIDELINES FOR TREATMENT OF MITRAL VALVE STENOSIS[29].

Asymptomatic patients
In the a-symptomatic patient, the severity of the stenosis measured with Doppler echocardiography determines the further steps to be taken. If the mitral valve area is
> 1.5 cm^2 and the mean gradient < 5 mmHg, no further evaluation is needed. It takes decades before progression occurs requiring intervention[35]. Follow-up consists of a yearly visit with a history and physical examination. A new echocardiogram is required if symptoms develop or the physical exam changes (fig 4).
If mitral valve area is < 1.5 cm^2 and gradient > 5 mmHg, the decision to proceed should be based on valve morphology and the effect of mitral stenosis on the pulmonary circulation. If the valve morphology is suitable for commisurotomy and there is a systolic pulmonary artery pressure > 50 mmHg, percutaneous balloon valvulotomy should be considered. If valve morphology is suitable for commisurotomy and pulmonary pressure is low, pulmonary pressures should be measured again after stress testing. If patients are not able to achieve adequate work load, become symptomatic and show elevation of the transmitral gradient or and a pulmonary artery pressure > 60 mmHg, further intervention should be considered.

10

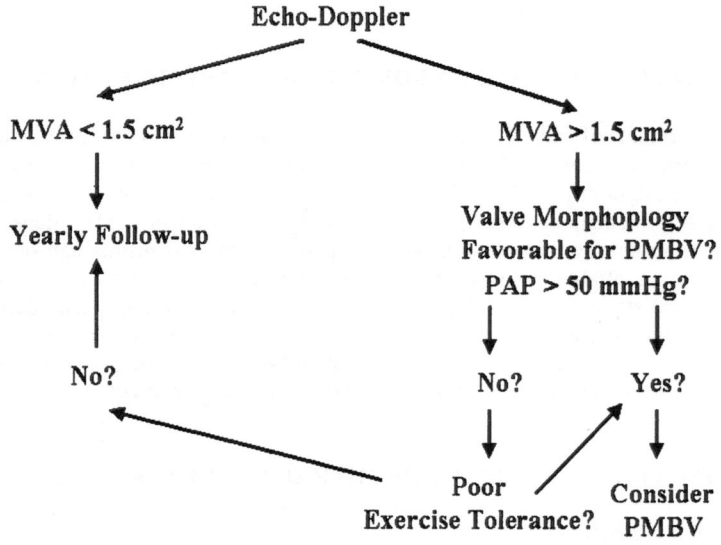

Figure 4: *Algorithm for the evaluation of patients with a-symptomatic mitral stenosis.*
PMVB = Percutaneous mitral balloon valvulotomy; MVA = mitral valve area;
PAP = pulmonary artery systolic pressure (From ACC/AHA Guidelines for Valvular Heart Disease[29].

Patients with class II symptoms
In patients with class 2 symptoms, a mitral valve area < 1.5 cm^2 and a gradient > 5 mmHg, the decision to proceed has to be based on mitral valve morphology (fig 5). If patients have a valve suitable for commissurotomy, percutaneous mitral balloon valvulotomy has to be performed. If the mitral valve area is > 1.5 cm^2 and the mean gradient < 5 mmHg exercise testing should be performed to determine if symptoms are due to the mitral stenosis.

Those patients, who have a significant rise in mean gradient with exercise and a pliable valve are candidates for mitral valve valvuloplasty.

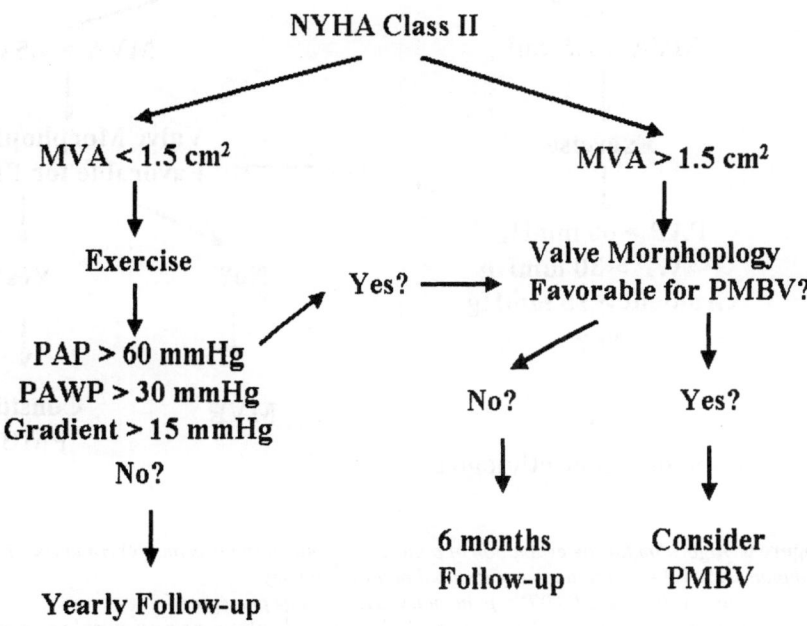

Figure 5: *Algorithm for the evaluation of patients with mitral stenosis and NYHA class II symptoms. PMVB = Percutaneous mitral balloon valvulotomy; MVA = mitral valve area; PAWP = pulmonary artery wedge pressure; PAP = pulmonary artery systolic pressure (From ACC/AHA Guidelines for Valvular Heart Disease[29].*

Patients with class III – IV symptoms
Patients with mitral stenosis and class III – IV symptoms have a poor prognosis if left untreated[4]. Therefore these patients have to be treated with either percutaneous balloon valvulotomy, mitral valve repair or mitral valve replacement.

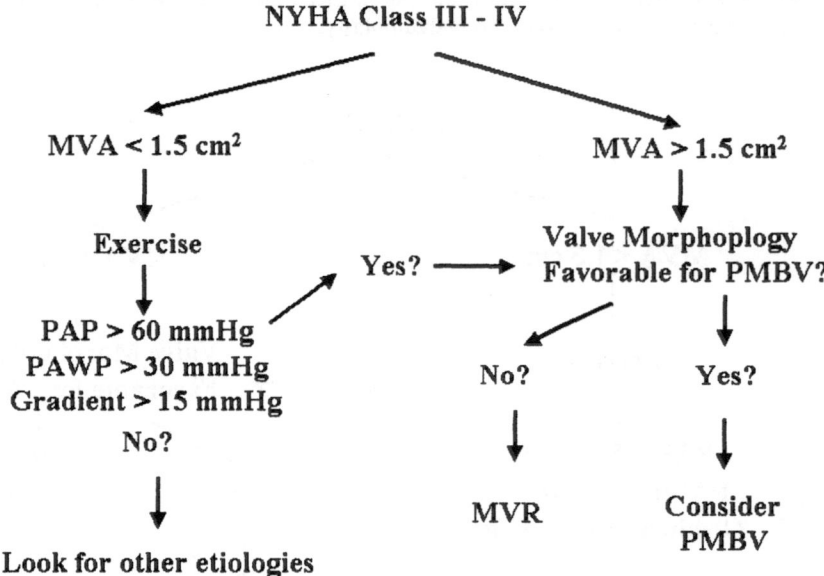

Figure 6: *Algorithm for the evaluation of patients with mitral stenosis and NYHA class III –IV symptoms. PMVB = Percutaneous mitral balloon valvulotomy; MVA = mitral valve area; PAWP = pulmonary artery wedge pressure; PAP = pulmonary artery systolic pressure; MVR = mitral valve repair or mitral valve replacement. (From ACC/AHA Guidelines for Valvular Heart Disease[29].*

REFERENCES

1. Rowe JC, Bland EF, Sprague HB. The course of mitral stenosis without surgery: ten and twenty year perspectives. Ann Intern Med 1960;52:741-749.
2. Roberts WC, Perloff JK. Mitral valvular disease: a clinicopathologic survey of the conditions causing the mitral valve to function abnormally. Ann Intern Med 1972;77:939-975.
3. Gorlin R, Gorlin S: Hydraulic formula for calculation of the area of stenotic mitral valve, other cardiac values and central circulatory shunts. Am. Heart J. 1951; 41: 1-29
4. Olesen K. The natural history of 271 patients with mitral stenosis under medical treatment. Br. Heart J. 1962; 24: 349-357.
5. Rowe J., Bland E., Sprague H.: the course of mitral stenosis without surgery: Ten and twenty year perspectives. Ann. Intern. Med. 1960; 52: 741-749.
6. Ward C, Hancock BW. Extreme pulmonary hypertension caused by mitral valve disease: natural history and results of surgery. Br Heart J 1975;37:74-78.
7. Wood P: An appreciation of mitral stenosis: Part I and part II. Br. Med. J. 1954; 1: 1051-1063, 1113-1124.
8. Reichek N., Shelburne J., Perfoff J.: Clinical aspects of rheumatic valvular disease. Prog. Cardiovasc. Dis. 1973; 15: 491-537.
9. Reis RN, Roberts WC.: Amounts of coronary arterial narrowing by atherosclerotic plaques in clinically isolated mitral valve stenosis: Analysis of 76 necropsy patients older than 30 years. Am. J. Cardiol. 1986; 57: 1117-1123.
10. Martin RP, Rakowski H, Kleiman JH, Beaver W, London E, Popp RL. Reliability and reproducibility of two dimensional echocardiographic measurement of the stenotic mitral valve orifice area. Am J Cardiol 1979;43:560-568.
11. Hatle L, Brubakk A, Tromsdal A, Angelsen B. Noninvasive assessment of pressure drop in mitral stenosis by Doppler ultrasound. Br Heart J 1978;40:131-140.
12. Fatkin D, Roy P, Morgan JJ, Feneley MP. Percutaneous balloon mitral valvotomy with the Inoue single-balloon catheter: commissural morphology as a determinant of outcome. J Am Coll Cardiol 1993;21:390-397.
13. Henry WL, Griffith JM, Michaelis LL, McIntosh CL, Morrow AG, Epstein SE. Measurement of mitral orifice area in patients with mitral valve disease by real-time, two-dimensional echocardiography. Circulation 1975;51:827-831.
14. Hugenholtz P., Ryan T., Stein S. the spectrum of pure mitral stenosis: Hemodynamic studies in relation to clinical disability. Am. J. Cardiol. 1962; 10: 773-784.
15. Hatle L, Angelsen B, Tromsdal A. Noninvasive assessment of atrioventricular pressure half-time by Doppler ultrasound. Circulation 1979;60:1096-1104.
16. Nakatani S, Masuyama T, Kodama K, Kitabatake A, Fujii K, Kamada T. Value and limitations of Doppler echocardiography in the quantification of stenotic mitral valve area: comparison of the pressure half-time and the continuity equation methods. Circulation 1988;77:78-85.
17. Thomas JD, Wilkins GT, Choong CY, et al. Inaccuracy of mitral pressure half-time immediately after percutaneous mitral valvotomy: dependence on transmitral gradient and left atrial and ventricular compliance. Circulation 1988;78:980-993.
18. Nakatani S., Masuyama T., Kodama K., Kitabatake A, Fujii K, Kamada T. Value and limitations of Doppler echocardiography in the qualification of stenotic mitral valve area: Comparison of the pressure half-time and the continuity equation methods. Circulation 1988; 77: 78-85.
19. Currie PJ, Seward JB, Chan KL, et al. Continuous wave Doppler determination of right ventricular pressure: a simultaneous Doppler-catheterization study in 127 patients. J Am Coll Cardiol 1985;6:750-756.

14

20. Leavitt JI, Coats MH, Falk RH. Effects of exercise on transmitral gradient and pulmonary artery pressure in patients with mitral stenosis or a prosthetic mitral valve: a Doppler echocardiographic study. J Am Coll Cardiol 1991;17:1520-1526.
21. Himelman RB, Stulbarg M, Kircher B, et al. Noninvasive evaluation of pulmonary artery pressure during exercise by saline-enhanced Doppler echocardiography in chronic pulmonary disease. Circulation 1989;79:863-871.
22. Alpert J The lessons of history as reflected In the pulmonary capillary wedge pressure. J. Am. Coll. Cardiol. 1989; 13: 830-831.
23. Nishimura R, Rihal C, Tajik A, et al Accurate measurement of the transmitral gradient in patients with mitral stenosis: A simultaneous catheterization and Doppler echocardiographic study. J. Am. Coll. Cardiol. 1994; 24: 152-158.
24. Reyes VP, Raju BS, Wynne J, et al. Percutaneous balloon valvuloplasty compared with open surgical commissurotomy for mitral stenosis. N Engl J Med 1994;331:961-967.
25. Ben Farhat M, Ayari M, Maatouk F, et al. Percutaneous balloon versus surgical closed and open mitral commissurotomy: seven-year follow-up results of a randomized trial. Circulation 1998;97:245-250.
26. Cohen DJ, Kuntz RE, Gordon SP, et al. Predictors of long-term outcome after percutaneous balloon mitral valvuloplasty. N Engl J Med 1992;327:1329-1335.
27. Complications, and mortality of percutaneous balloon mitral commissurotomy: a report from the National Heart, Lung, and Blood Institute Balloon Valvuloplasty Registry. Circulation 1992;85:2014-2024.
28. Wilkins GT, Weyman A, Abascal VM, Block PC, Palacios IF. Percutaneous balloon dilatation of the mitral valve: an analysis of echocardiographic variables related to outcome and the mechanism of dilatation. Br. Heart J. 1988; 60: 299-308.
29. Bonow et al, ACC/AHA Task Force Report: Management of Patients with Valvular Heart Disease J Am Coll Cardiol 1998; 32: 1486-588
30. Palacios IF, Tuzcu ME, Weyman AE, Newell JB, Block PC. Clinical follow-up of patients undergoing percutaneous mitral balloon valvotomy. Circulation 1995;91:671– 676.
31. Dean LS, Mickel M, Bonan R, et al. Four-year follow-up of patients undergoing percutaneous balloon mitral commissurotomy: a report from the National Heart, Lung, and Blood Institute Balloon Valvuloplasty Registry. J Am Coll Cardiol 1996;28:1452–1457.
32. Cannan CR, Nishimura RA, Reeder GS, et al. Echocardiographic assessment of commissural calcium: a simple predictor of outcome after percutaneous mitral balloon valvotomy. J Am Coll Cardiol 1997;29:175–180.
33. Bruce J, Nishimura R. Clinical assessment and management of mitral stenosis. Cardiology Clinics 1998; 16: 375-403.
34. Longo M, Previti A, Morello M., Greco O., Decio A., Pansini S., Morea M., Mangiardi ML. Usefulness of transesophageal echocardiography during open heart surgery of mitral stenosis. J Cardiovasc. Surg. 2000; 41: 381-385.
35. Selzer A, Cohn K. Natural history of mitral stenosis: a review. Circulation 1972; 45: 878-890.

Section I / Chapter 2

PREOPERATIVE EVALUATION OF MITRAL REGURGITATION: THE CHALLENGE OF OPTIMAL TIMING

C.H. PEELS

INTRODUCTION

Mitral regurgitation (MR) results in sole volume overload of the left ventricle, with the increased volume pumped into the systemic circulation as well as in the low-impedance left atrium. This results in a an increase in pre-load of the left ventricle and a decrease in afterload.

In acute MR the left ventricle compensates for the sudden increase in preload by increasing the diastolic sarcomere length thus the diastolic volume and this leads to increase in stroke work. The ejection of blood through the incompetent mitral valve into the low-resistance left atrium accounts for the decrease in afterload. This augments left ventricular emptying and thus leads to a an increase in ejection fraction and a decrease in end-systolic volume.

When MR becomes chronic from this stage on or increases in severity slowly, this volume overload situation leads to left ventricular enlargement and compensatory eccentric hypertrophy resulting in an increase in left ventricular volume and mass: the radius of the left ventricle increases without a significant change in wall thickness. Wall stress thus stays or returns within the normal range.

The increased enddiastolic volume enables augmentation of total stroke volume and maintenance of forward stroke volume within the normal range. Compared to acute MR, where emptying of the left ventricle is augmented, in chronic MR the ejection fraction stays in the compensated phase within the normal range. Transition to the decompensated phase is characterized by declination of contractile function, a situation which can be prevented by optimal timing of surgical intervention.

In the evaluation of patients with MR, besides assessment of the cause and severity of MR, most crucial for timing of surgery is the assessment of left ventricular function.

These aspects will be dealt with in this order and furthermore the question why timing is so essential is highlighted. The factors inducing a shift to more early surgical intervention than the classical point where patients become symptomatic, will be elucidated thereafter.

EVALUATION OF THE CAUSE OF MR

Mitral valve repair as the treatment of severe MR has been shown to render operative and long-term survival advantages over mitral valve replacement, partly ascribed to the preservation of left ventricular geometry. Because of this potential of mitral valve repair, revealing the specific anatomic or functional defect responsible for regurgitation is essential to uncover those valves with ability to be repaired. This requests close cooperation between the cardiologist and the surgeon to understand the described valve pathology on one hand and to know the surgical possibilities on the other hand.

More certain prediction whether a valve can be repaired favors more early surgical intervention. The lack of the drawbacks of a prosthetic valve allow us to focus on the need to obviate the occult development of myocardial contractile dysfunction and intervene at the earliest sign of ventricular or even atrial dysfunction. Whether this should be done in asymptomatic patients is not recommended in literature and is an ideal question to be answered in a randomized trial.

Since mitral valve closure results from the complex interaction of each of the components of the valve apparatus, MR evolves from alterations in one of these components: the left atrial wall, the annulus, the leaflets, the chordae, the papillary muscles and the left ventricular wall.

Although left atrial dilation typically is the result rather than the cause of MR, progressive atrial enlargement due to chronic atrial fibrillation can lead to annular dilation and progressive MR[1], a condition suitable for valve repair.

Mitral annular calcification is seen mostly between the posterior leaflet of the mitral valve and the left ventricular myocardium. Although it is usually functionally insignificant, it can lead to valve dysfunction, most frequent MR, caused by interference with annular contraction during systole or by failure of leaflet coaptation. Whether repair can lead to a competent valve is uncertain.

Impairment of the mitral leaflets and chordae is most commonly nowadays caused by myxomatous degenerative disease, rheumatic affliction of valve leaflets as the cause of MR has decreased in the last 20 years to around 3 percent in some series of surgical patients[2,3].

Success of valve repair depends upon the amount of valve tissue affected, affliction of the anterior leaflet, certainly when it is more than one third of the leaflet surface, signifies limited possibilities for repair. Annular dilation often is present in patients with myxomatous valve disease implying annuloplasty as part of the repair.

Infectious endocarditis is a significant cause of MR. Preoperative evaluation is focused on detection of vegetations, indicating the size of them and elucidating the complications of valve destruction as perforation of leaflets, deformity of the coaptation zone, rupture of chordae or loss of normal annular and commissural support structures. Furthermore attention has to be payed to complications as paravalvular abcess and fistula formation. MR onset in these patients usually is sudden and poorly tolerated when severe thus leading to urgent surgery because of hemodynamic deterioration. Depending on the stage of the infectious disease in which the patient has to be operated and the degree of valve tissue destruction valve repair can be done.

Ischemic MR accounts for a large amount of patients undergoing mitral valve surgery, around 30 percent[4]. Papillary muscle rupture caused by a localized transmural infarction leads to catastrophic acute MR due to partial or complete rupture of the muscle, is rare (<0,1% of infarct patients) but has to be recognized immediately to ensure quick intervention. Mortality rate without surgery is extremely high, around 95% within 2 weeks, and valve replacement is usually needed. Operative mortality still is high, averaging 50% in most series, but intervention can be life saving in appropriately selected patients concerning comorbid disease, ventricular function and clinical status.

Significant MR without abnormalities of the valve leaflets or annular dimensions is seen in acute myocardial infarction due to alterations in regional left ventricular function and shape[5]. Most often the infarction is located in the flow area of the right or circumflex coronary artery and is associated with inferior wall motion abnormalities[6]. On 2 DE the posterior leaflet slides under the anterior and a MR jet is directed anteriorly. The effect of reperfusion on these ischemic MR's remains controversial and depends on the mechanism of MR: when annular dilation associated with inferior wall motion abnormalities is present, reperfusion alone is not enough to achieve valve competence and annuloplasty is needed[4, 7, 8].

MR commonly occurs in patients with left ventricular dilation and systolic dysfunction, whether this results from end-stage ischemic disease or dilated cardiomyopathy of any cause. The valve leaflets and chordae are structurally normal but the 3D anatomic relationships of the valve apparatus components are distorted leading to incompetence. Typically, regurgitant severity can be altered dramatically in response to altering loading conditions. This MR may respond favorably to vasodilator therapy with even improvement in ejection performance[9]. Benefit from surgical placement of an annuloplasty ring despite severe systolic dysfunction is suggested by some[10].

EVALUATION OF THE SEVERITY OF MR

Obviously, patients should not undergo valve surgery unless there is severe regurgitation. Non-invasive imaging can provide all the information needed to gauge the severity of MR: left and right ventricular function, the cause and severity of MR, the presence of pulmonary hypertension and associated valve lesions as tricuspid regurgitation and aortic valve disease.. Cardiac catheterisation with exercise hemodynamics and angiography is only indicated when there is discrepancy between clinical and non-invasive findings. Although ventriculography has its own limitations[11], it provides an additional method to assess chamber dilation and function and to estimate MR severity. Right heart catheterisation is only indicated when there is uncertainty about MR severity and pulmonary hypertension. Coronary angiography is indicated in patients with risk factors for coronary artery disease including age, hypercholesterolemia, and hypertension.

When in acute MR, severe regurgitation is suspected from the clinical indices, a patient in pulmonary edema and cardiogenic shock, simple non-invasive findings can immediately confirm this suspicion : 2D echocardiography shows a left ventricle 'to good' for this clinical situation with a decreased endsystolic volume and a high ejection fraction and color flow Doppler shows the regurgitant jet in the left atrium, often eccentric. For adequate imaging of the latter and good visualisation of the cause of MR, transesophageal echocardiography is often superior above transthoracic imaging in this situation[12].

Also in chronic MR, severity is indicated by the changes in left ventricular dimension but also by left atrial dimensions: both are enlarged. In severe MR, the enddiastolic dimension of the left ventricle increases as a response to volume overload without significant increase in wall thickness because afterload stays more or less the same. The endsystolic dimension indicates not only severity of regurgitation but above all the contractile state of the myocardium. In contrast to acute MR where a depressed ejection fraction and an increased systolic volume precludes possible other reasons for the cardiogenic shock than pure acute MR, in chronic MR this points out contractile dysfunction induced by prolonged severe MR.

Grading of severity should be done by integrating the data from 2D imaging of valve and ventricles and Doppler measures. Semi-quantitative grading can be done non-invasively using color flow imaging generating length, height, area of the color flow jet and the width of the vena contracta, pulsed Doppler transvalvular velocities and flow measures in the pulmonary veins and continuous wave Doppler measures. Traditionally, grading is done in a 4-point scale:

0   = none
1+ = mild; disturbed flow localized to the region immediately adjacent to mitral
     valve closure, may not be seen in every beat, consistent with normal or
     physiologic regurgitation.
2+ = mild to moderate; disturbed flow filling up to one third of the cross sectional
     area of the left atrium, seen on every beat
3+ = moderate to severe; disturbed flow filling up to two thirds of the cross sectional
     area of the left atrium, seen on every beat
4+ = severe; disturbed flow almost filling the cross sectional area of the left atrium,
     systolic flow reversal in the pulmonary veins

The assigned grade is based on two orthogonal planes and integration of the extent of flow disturbance in both views[13].

Signal attenuation from the apical views may lead to underestimation of regurgitant severity, especially in the presence of prosthetic mitral valves. Transesophageal imaging allows optimization of the regurgitant color flow image; the physician needs to be aware of the effects of depth, pulse repetition frequency and transducer frequency that can lead to differences in jet size with transthoracic imaging[14].

For grading MR severity in terms of quantification, several new approaches have been proposed: calculation of flow rates from the proximal convergence zone (also known as the PISA method), momentum quantification in the regurgitant jet and calculation of the regurgitant orifice area (ROA)[15]. Quantifying the ROA is theoretically the best fundamental measure of valve abnormality and will likely evolve as one of the principal indices of regurgitation.

$$ROA = (area\ of\ jet\ x\ V^2\ jet\ )\ /\ V^2 orifice$$

V jet is measured with pulsed Doppler at any downstream site of the color flow jet
Vorifice is measured with continuous wave Doppler in the orifice.

Color flow indices and regurgitant fraction vary with the transvalvular driving pressure and thus give information not only on the regurgitation but also on the stroke volume which can be affected by long standing regurgitation. On the contrary, ROA reflects the real abnormality of the valve although it may change with changing loading conditions but these are real changes in the valve lesion. Untill now, it was and still is impractical to measure and it is not yet validated sufficiently.

Indirect markers of severity of regurgitation are the mitral inflow and pulmonary venous flow pattern obtained with pulsed wave doppler.

For follow-up those indices should be chosen which are reliably obtainable and are reproducible in the hands of the clinician.

LEFT VENTRICULAR FUNCTION AND MITRAL REGURGITATION

It is generally accepted that MR places relatively favorable loading conditions on the left ventricle, because the low impedance leak during systole allows maintenance of a high normal ejection fraction (EF) and even when contractility is depressed, a low normal EF can be maintained[16].

However, after mitral valve replacement or even after mitral valve repair, left ventricular function tends to fall postoperatively[17], even when it was within the normal range pre-operatively. Patients with chronic MR are followed closely to prevent left ventricular dysfunction to occur and several markers are used to indicate the early development of this unfavorable development. That chronic overload depresses the myocardial contractile state eventually has been deduced from clinical observations but never directly proven. Whether this depressed performance can be attributed to chronic volume overload per se or to an associated condition such as rheumatic myocarditis or other cardiomyopathies is not certain. The last conditions could explain why in some patients with chronic MR after mitral valve surgery contractile dysfunction develops depite normal function preoperatively[18]. When there is marked increase in left ventricular size preoperatively, even when function is only minimally depressed, postoperatively left ventricular function can deteriorate further in 6 to 12 months.

This 'silent' dysfunction of the left ventricle can not be detected easily, but increase in volume and decrease in ejection fraction can. These are the parameters to follow in patients with chronic MR and guidelines have been made to decide for surgery in the still asymptomatic patient[19]. When echocardiographic parameters as endsystolic dimension (ESD)and EF indicate left ventricular dysfunction, ESD $\geq$ 45 mm and EF $\leq$ 0.60, mitral valve surgery is indicated. Surgery is always indicated in the symptomatic patient with severe MR, even when these indices point out a still normal left ventricular function (ESD < 45 mm and EF > 0.60).

In view of the above mentioned observation that normal preoperative left ventricular function can belie the true contractile state and surprise the physician with a depressed left ventricular function and therefore still symptomatic patient after surgery, repair of a severely regurgitant valve may be contemplated even in an asymptomatic patient with a normal left ventricular function and dimensions in order to preserve the ventricular function present at that moment. Of course, prediction of likelihood of repair should be as accurate as possible and performance of the repair should be done in centers where the successfulness is high.

WHY OPTIMAL TIMING

Aware of the difficulty of detecting the onset of contractile dysfunction, this could serve as a stimulus for earlier referral for surgery when severe MR is diagnosed. However, there are two major reasons to strive for optimal timing: firstly, the morbidity but moreover the mortality associated with valve surgery and secondly the disadvantages of the possession of a valve prosthesis.

Mitral valve surgery still has substantial mortality, replacement having a higher short and long-term mortality rate than repair. Operative mortality for replacement is 3-29% with an average of 5-10%, and long-term survival is relatively poor, rates between 50 and 85%[20], with improvement in later series. Mortality rates for mitral valve repair are lower, hospital mortality being 1-10%.

Mitral valve repair and mitral valve replacement with preservation of the chordal apparatus not only lead to better preservation of ventricular function than replacement[21] with severed chordae but also to better survival[22].

Nevertheless, the possession of a prosthetic valve, a situation which can always occur even when repair is planned, introduces valve-related morbidity and mortality, so called 'prosthetic valve disease', the most important being thrombo-embolic events (a risk around 0.6-2,3% per patient year), and anti coagulation related hemorrhage and a higher susceptibility to endocarditis. Although valve repair obviates the need for anticoagulation when sinus rhythm is still present and thus prevents hemorrhagic complications and has a almost negligible risk for late endocarditis, failed repair would still result in a prosthetic valve most of the time.

Hence, optimal timing is still necessary in the asymptomatic patient with severe MR and prophylactic surgery not recommended.

FACTORS INFLUENCING TIMING OF SURGERY

Several variables have been described to influence outcome after surgery for severe MR. Besides echocardiographic variables, these include age, functional class >I, presence of coronary artery disease [17,23] and hemodynamic variables as mean pulmonary artery pressure and cardiac index[24]. The echocardiographic markers indicating poor outcome were ESD >45-50mm[17, 23, 25] and EF < 50-60%[17,23]. One must be aware that these variables are derived from studies where they identified patients with poor outcome after surgery. So, in no way it is proven that they point out accurately the onset of occult left ventricular dysfunction still being reversible. In this respect, is a significant change from baseline of ESD and EF a much stronger indicator of the onset of contractile dysfunction and should lead to prompt referral for surgery, than the reaching of the values of the absolute parameters per se. The values mentioned are only indications for patients who are asymptomatic and seen for the first time.

Symptomatic patients with severe MR always should be referred for surgery, especially when there are signs of heart failure, decreased exercise tolerance or atrial arrhythmias such as atrial fibrillation. One should be very meticulous in detecting these symptoms especially in patients with long existing mitral regurgitation because these patients are used to a slowly decreasing exercise tolerance; exercise testing is a good tool in these patients follow-up.

The recent experiences with mitral valve repair even in patients with severe systolic dysfunction of the left ventricle suggests that this referral should take place even in these patients[26].However, when valve repair is not feasible, mitral valve replacement should be considered only with extreme caution because high operative mortality and a very poor long-term outcome exists in these patients because left ventricular function most likely further deteriorates after surgery.

22

REFERENCES

1. Tanimoto M, Pai RG: Effect of isolated left atrial enlargement on mitral annular size and valve
2. competence. Am J Cardiol 1996; 77: 769-774
3. Cosgrove DM, Stewart WJ: Mitral valvuloplasty, Curr Probl Cardiol 1989; 14: 359-415
4. Loop FD, Cosgrove DM, Stewart WJ: Mitral valve repair for mitral insufficiency. Eur Heart J 1991; 12S: 30-33
5. Rankin JS, Hickey MS, Smith LR et al: Ischemic mitral regurgitation. Circulation 1989; 79: 16-21
6. van Dantzig JM, Delemarre BJ, Koster RW, Bot H, Visser CA;Pathogenesis of mitral regurgitation in acute myocardial infarction: importance of changes in left ventriculra shape and regional function. Am Heart J 1996;131:865-871
7. Sharma SK, Seckler J, Israel DH, Borrico S, Ambrose JA: Clinical, angiographic and anatomic findings in acute severe ischemic mitral regurgitation. Am J Cardiol 1992;70:277-280
8. Kaul S, Spotnitz WD, Glasheen WP, Touchstone DA: Mechanism of ischemic mitral regurgitation: an experimental evaluation. Circulation 1991;84:2167-2180
9. Kay GL, Kay JH, Zubiate P, Yokoyama T, Mendez M: Mitral valve repair for mitral regurgitation secondary to coronary artery disease. Circulation 1986;74:88-98
10. Evangelista MA, Bruguera CJ, Serrat SR, et al: Influence of mitral regurgitation on the response to captopril therapy for congestive heart failure caused by idiopathic dilated cardiomyopathy. Am J Cardiol 1992;69:373-376
11. Bach DS, Bolling SF: Early improvement in congestive heart failure after correction of secondary mitral regurgitation in end-stage cardiomyopathy. Am Heart J 1995;129: 1165-1170
12. Croft CH, Lipscomb K, Mathis K et al. Limitations of qualitative angiographic grading in aortic and mitral regurgitation. Am J Cardiol 1984;53:1593-1598
13. Manning JW, Wakmonski CA, Boyle NG: Papillary muscle rupture complicating inferior myocardial infarction: identification with transesophageal echocardiography. Am Heart J 1995;129:191-193
14. Spain MG, Smith MD, Grayburn PA, Harlamert EA, DeMaria AN: Quantitative assessment of mitral regurgitation by Doppler   color flow imaging: angiographic and hemodynamic correlations. J Am Coll Cardiol 1989;13:585-590
15. Smith MD, Harrison MR, Pinton R, Kandil H, Kwan OL, DeMaria AN: Regurgitant jet size by transesophageal compared with   transthoracic Doppler color flow imaging. Circulation 1991;83:79-86
16. Vandervoort PM, Thomas JD; New approaches to qauntification of valvular regurgitation. In Otto CM, ed. The practice of clinical echocardiography. Philadelphia: WB Saunders, 1997:307-326.
17. Ross Jr J: Left ventricular function and timing of surgical treatment in valvular heart disease. Ann Intern Med 1981;94:498-504
18. Enriquez-Sarano M, Tajik AJ, Schaff HV et al: Echocardiographic prediction of left ventricular function after correction of mitral regurgitation: results and clinical implications. J Am Coll Cardiol 1994;24:1536-1543
19. Starling MR, Kirsh MM, Montgomery DG, Gross MD: Impaired left ventricular contractile function in patients with long-term mitral regurgitation and normal ejection fraction. J Am Coll Cardiol 1993;22:239-250

20. Bonow RO, Carabello B, de Leon AC Jr, Edmunds LH Jr, Fedderly BJ, Freed MD, Gaasch WH, McKay CR, Nishimura RA, O'Gara PR, O'Rourke RA, Rahimtoola SH. ACC/AHA Guidelines for the management of patients with valvular heart disease: a report of the American College of Cardiology/American Heart Association Task Force on Practice Guidelines (Committee on
21. management of patients with valvualr heart disease). J Am Coll Cardiol 1998;32:1486-1588
22. Lindblom D, Lindblom U, Qvist J, Lundstrom H: Long-term survival rates after heart valve replacement. J Am Coll Cardiol 1990;15:566-573
23. Rozich JD, Carabello BA, Usher BW, Kratz JM, Bell AE, Zile MR: Mitral valve replacement with and without chordal preservation in patients with chronic mitral regurgitation: mechanisms for differences in postoperative ejection performance. Circulation 1992;86:1718-1726
24. Lee EM, Shapiro LM, Wells FC: Importance of subvalvular preservation and early operation in mitral valve surgery. Circulation 1996;94:2117-2123
25. Enriquez-Sarano M, Tajik AJ, Schaff HV et al: Echocardiographic prediction of survival after surgical correction of organic mitral regurgitation. Circulation 1994;90:830-837
26. Crawford MH, Souchek J, Oprian CA, Miller DC, Rahimtoola S, Giacomini JC, Sethi G, Hammermeister KE; Determinants of survival and left ventricular performance after mitral valve replacement. Circulation 1990;81:1173-1181
27. Wisenbaugh T, Skudicky D, Sareli P: Prediction of outcome after valve replacement for rheumatic mitral regurgitation in the era of chordal preservation. Circulation 1994;89:191-197
28. Bach DS, Bolling SF: Early improvement in congestive heart failure after correction of secondary mitral regurgiatation in end-stage cardiomyopathy. Am Heart J 1995;129:1165-1170

Section 1 / Chapter 3

PERIOPERATIVE TRANSESOPHAGEAL ECHOCARDIOGRAPHY IN MITRAL VALVE SURGERY

Dr. R.B.A. VAN DEN BRINK, Prof.Dr. B.A.J.M. DE MOL

INTRODUCTION

Mitral valve repair seems to offer important advantages over valve replacement with less mortality and morbidity[1]. Therefore patients requiring surgical intervention for mitral regurgitation are increasingly undergoing mitral valve reconstruction rather than mitral valve replacement. However, mitral valve repair is often technically more demanding than valve replacement. Optimal results of mitral valve repair require the surgeon to understand the mechanism of mitral regurgitation. Multiplane TransEsophageal Echocardiography (TEE) provides an ideal tool to obtain information on the mechanism and severity of mitral regurgitation.

As to mitral valve repair, the present review will address the following topics:
- How to visualize the mechanism of mitral valve regurgitation by multiplane TEE?
- How to assess severity of mitral regurgitation?
- Does intraoperative TEE during mitral valve repair predict early and late mitral valve dysfunction?
  - Pitfalls in the intraoperative assessment of the severity of mitral regurgitation.
  - What extent of mitral regurgitation assessed by intraoperative TEE will allow satisfactory late results?
  - Complications after mitral valve repair

If mitral valve repair is not possible, mitral valve replacement is performed. All mechanical valves and most bioprosthetic valves are obstructive to flow and have a closure and leakage backflow pattern that is dependent on the prosthetic valve design. In order to be able to recognize prosthetic valve dysfunction, it is important to be familiar with the Doppler echocardiographic characteristics of various normally functioning prosthetic valves.

As far as mitral valve replacement is concerned the present review will address:

- The Doppler echocardiographic flow characteristics of several types of normally functioning mitral prosthetic valves.
- Characteristics and causes of pathologic obstruction or leakage of mitral valve prostheses.

HOW TO IMAGE THE MECHANISM OF MITRAL VALVE REGURGITATION BY MULTIPLANE TEE?

The mitral valve is composed of the anterior and posterior leaflets, chordae tendinae, papillary muscles, annulus and left ventricular walls. All these parts should be visualized by TEE to get an impression of the mitral valve function and the mechanism of mitral regurgitation.

Obviously, to obtain an optimal result of mitral valve repair it is necessary for the cardiac surgeon and echocardiographer to understand each other.

ANATOMY OF THE MITRAL VALVE: THE SURGEONS VIEW
(figure 1)

The surgeon inspecting the mitral valve from the left atrium views the lateral commissure to his left and the medial commissure to his right. The posterior mitral leaflet has three scallops: the anterolateral (P1), middle (P2) and posteromedial (P3) scallop. The left part of the middle scallop possesses chordal attachments to the anterolateral papillary muscle and the right part to the posteromedial papillary muscle. The anterior mitral leaflet has no scallops and is divided in an anterolateral part (A1), a middle part (A2) and a posteromedial part (A3). The anterior and posterior halves of the anterior mitral leaflet have chordal attachments to the anterolateral and posteromedial papillary muscle respectively.

THE ECHOCARDIOGRAPHERS VIEW

The mitral valve is examined by using 4 mid-esophageal views and 3 transgastric views[2]. It is important in all planes to maximize left ventricular cavity size in order to transect the mitral orifice at its centre. In the mid esophageal views this often requires some retroflexion of the probe tip. Depending on the position of the heart in relation to the esophagus the angles to visualize certain parts of the mitral valve may vary somewhat in individual patients.

First the anatomical structures of the mitral valve are visualized and thereafter the entire sequence of views is repeated in the Color Doppler flow imaging mode.

Mid esophageal views (transducer depth 30-40 cm from the incisors). See figure I.

The 'four chamber view' (both atria and both ventricles) is obtained at a multiplane angle of 0^0 - 20^0 and displays the middle section of the anterior mitral leaflet (A2) at the left of the image display and the middle scallop of the posterior mitral leaflet (P2) to the right.

Sometimes the anterolateral scallop of the posterior mitral leaflet (P1) instead of P2 is displayed in this view.

The 'mitral-commissural view' is obtained at 60^0 - 70^0. This view displays the anterior mitral leaflet in the middle of the image, the anterolateral commissure and anterolateral scallop of the posterior leaflet (P1) to the right and the posteromedial commissure and posteromedial scallop of the posterior mitral leaflet (P3) to the left of the image.

1. The 'two-chamber view' (left atrium and left ventricle) is obtained at 90^0. This view displays the posteromedial scallop of the posterior mitral valve leaflet (P3) to the left and the anterolateral part of the anterior mitral leaflet (A1) to the right.

2. The 'long-axis view' (left atrium, left ventricle and aorta) is obtained at 120^0 - 160^0. This view displays the middle scallop of the posterior mitral valve leaflet (P2) to the left and the middle part of the anterior mitral leaflet (A2) at the right.

   Transgastric views (transducer depth 40-50 cm from the incisors).

3. The transgastric 'mid short-axis view' is visualized at 0^0 - 20^0. In this view the posteromedial papillary muscle is displayed to the upper left and the anterolateral papillary muscle to the lower right. The papillary muscles are situated below the commissures of the mitral valve. In this view, wall motion abnormalities in left ventricular segments adjacent to the papillary muscles are detected.

4. The transgastric 'basal short-axis view' is also visualized at 0^0 - 20^0 by advancing the probe a little deeper in the stomach and anteflexing it with the big wheel. In this view the posteromedial commissure is displayed in the upper left of the image and the anterolateral commissure to the lower right, the anterior leaflet is to the left and the posterior leaflet to the right. This view gives the best impression of which part of the anterior and / or posterior leaflet is affected.

5. The transgastric basal 'two-chamber view' is obtained at the same level at 80^0 - 100^0 ; in this view chordae to the posteromedial papillary muscle are seen at the top of the image and chordae to the anterolateral papillary muscle to the bottom.

28

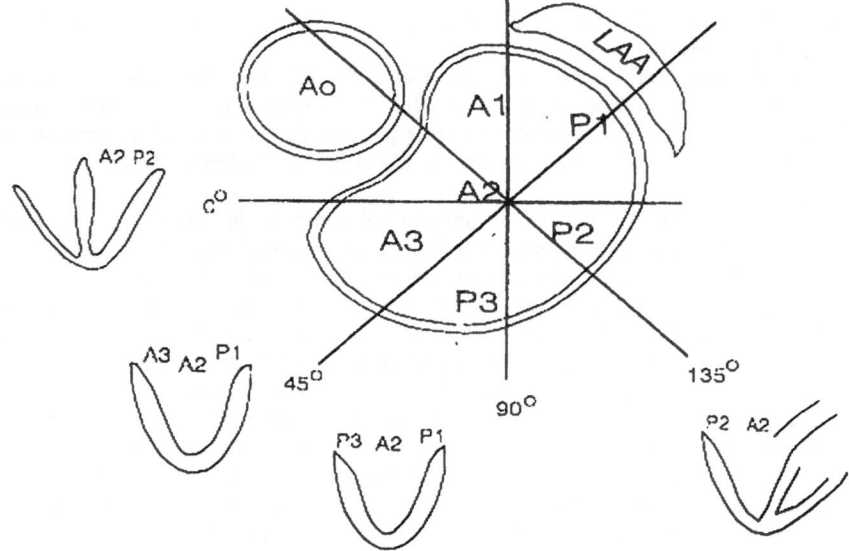

Figure I. *Mitral valve seen from the apex and midesophageal TEE imaging views*
Transverse view or 0 ⁰ ; bi-commisural view or 60 ⁰; longitudinal 'two chamber' view or 90 ⁰;
longaxis view or 135 ⁰.
A1 = anterolateral part of the anterior mitral valve leaflet (AMVL); A2 = middle part of the AMVL;
A3 = posteromedial part of the AMVL.
P 1 = anterolateral scallop of the posterior mitral valve leaflet (PMVL); P2 = middle scallop of the
PMVL; P3 = posteromedial scallop of the PMVL.
Reprinted with permission from the Society of Thoracic Surgeons. (The Annals of Thoracic Surgery
1998; 65: 1025-31 Foster GP et al.)

FUNCTION OF THE MITRAL VALVE

Mitral regurgitation may develop if one or more of the components of the mitral valve
(leaflets, chordae tendinae, papillary muscles, annulus, left ventricle) do not function
properly or demonstrate anatomic abnormalities. Using TEE the functional anatomy of the
mitral valve apparatus can be studied into detail.

Position of the mitral valve leaflets after closing
Normally the leaflets will close on the same level in the mitral annulus plane making
contact with each other along the closure line.

Malcoaptation of the leaflets exists if the leaflets are not in contact with each other after
closure. This may be caused by annular or ventricular dilatation and by commissural fusion
or shortening (scarring) of a leaflet.

Malapposition of the leaflets is present if the leaflets do not close at the same level. This is for instance the case if some chordae are elongated and the free edge of one of the leaflets overrides the annular plane. This situation in which the free edge of the prolapsing leaflet still is directed to the left ventricle is called a mitral valve prolapse. It has to be distinguished from a flail leaflet caused by chordal or papillary muscle rupture in which a part of the free edge of the mitral valve is floating freely in the left atrium. Malapposition is also present if one leaflet overrides the other leaflet because of retraction of that leaflet

Motion of the mitral valve leaflets
Normal leaflet motion. Normal leaflet motion is characterized by normal apposition and coaptation of the leaflets during systole and normal opening during diastole. In this case a leaflet perforation or congenital cleft may cause mitral regurgitation. The regurgitant jet does not originate at the coaptation line but at the base or body of the valve leaflets.
Excessive leaflet motion. Excessive leaflet motion occurs if chordae or a papillary muscle are elongated or ruptured. This leads to malapposition (prolapse) and/ or malcoaptation (flail leaflet). This mechanism of mitral regurgitation may be found in degenerative (myxomatous) mitral valve disease, papillary muscle infarction and endocarditis. The regurgitant jet is directed away from the most severely affected leaflet.
Restricted leaflet motion. Restricted leaflet motion is present if one or both leaflets do not open fully during diastole or if the body of one leaflet is hold back in the left ventricular cavity during systole at an unusual distance from the annular plane. Malapposition and /or malcoaptation of the leaflets may occur. This mechanism of mitral regurgitation is present in rheumatic valve disease, in papillary muscle infarction with shortening of the papillary muscle and segmental left ventricular asynergy. The regurgitant jet is directed towards the most severely affected valve leaflet.

Size of the annulus of the mitral valve
Annular dilatation can be measured by TEE in the mid esophageal long-axis view. In this view the antero-posterior annulus diameter can be measured from the hinge point between non-coronary cusp of the aortic valve and anterior mitral valve leaflet to the hinge point of the posterior mitral leaflet. This diameter should not be larger than 30 mm for small adults and not larger than 35 mm for normal adults.
Annular dilatation is often present in degenerative and in rheumatic mitral regurgitation. It may also be found in congestive cardiomyopathy if the left ventricle assumes a spherical shape instead of the normal ellipsoid one. This leads to outward displacement of the papillary muscles and to apical displacement of the closure line of the mitral valve leaflets toward the apex. The regurgitant jet is located centrally.

The extent of chordal elongation

The extent of chordal elongation in different segments of the mitral valve may be determined by measuring the extent of leaflet prolapse above the annular plane in the mid-oesophageal 4-chamber, 2-chamber and long-axis view. These measurements may provide to the surgeon an estimate of the extent of chordal shortening that is needed.

An overview of mechanisms of mitral regurgitation detectable with TEE and some of the repair techniques is shown in table 1.

MECHANISM OF MITRAL REGURGITATION BY TRANSESOPHAGEAL ECHOCARDIOGRAPHY AS COMPARED WITH SURGICAL FINDINGS

Several studies have demonstrated that multiplane TEE offers advantages in assessment of the mechanism and severity of mitral regurgitation over biplane (transverse 0-20^0 and longitudinal 70-110^0) TEE and biplane TEE is better than monoplane (only transverse plane) TEE[3,4,5].

Stewart et al[6]. assessed the accuracy of two-dimensional and dopplerechocardiography by multiplane TEE in determining the mechanism of mitral regurgitation as compared with direct inspection of the valve at operation by the surgeon. They studied 286 patients (60.2 ± 13.5 years) who underwent mitral valve repair over a 22 month interval.

The surgeon determined the mechanism of mitral regurgitation in the arrested heart by inspection of leaflets and annulus for redundancy, vegetations, perforations, fibrosis and calcifications. The chordae were inspected to determine the presence of chordal elongation, rupture, fibrosis, calcification or fusion and the papillary muscles for elongation, rupture or infarction. Leaflet motion was determined using a nerve hook and classified as follows: leaflet motion was restricted when maximal extension of the leaflet edge was on the left ventricular side of the annular plane. Leaflet motion was classified as normal when the leaflet edge was in the annular plane and excessive when the leaflet extended into the left atrial side of the mitral annulus.

In this study 7 different regurgitant mechanisms were distinguished, namely 1) posterior leaflet prolapse or flail; 2) anterior leaflet prolapse or flail; 3) bileaflet prolapse or flail; 4) papillary muscle elongation or disruption; 5) restricted leaflet motion; 6) ventricular-annular dilatation; and 7) leaflet perforation or cleft.

Agreement between surgical and echocardiographic findings was present in 93% of patients with posterior leaflet prolapse or flail, 94% with anterior leaflet prolapse or flail, and in 44% with bileaflet prolapse or flail. Surgical and echocardiographic findings were also in accordance in 75% of patients with papillary muscle elongation or disruption, 91% with restricted leaflet motion, 72% with ventricular-annular dilatation and 62% with leaflet perforation or cleft. Most frequent reasons for disagreement between surgical and TEE findings on the regurgitant mechanisms were: bileaflet prolapse at surgery classified as prolapse of only one leaflet by TEE, ventricular-annular dilatation by surgery classified as restricted leaflet motion by

TEE and leaflet perforation at surgery in patients in whom no regurgitant jet outside the coaptation line was seen by Doppler echocardiography.

The overall agreement between findings of the surgeon and the echocardiographer using TEE was 84%.

Grewal et al[7]. studied 54 patients with a flail mitral leaflet to assess the accuracy of TEE localization of the flail scallop as compared with findings at operation. They found an overall accuracy of 88%. The most common misdiagnosis was incorrect identification of a flail middle scallop of the PMVL (P2) as anterolateral (P1), because of visualization of the fail leaflet in the midesophageal view at 0^0. This is caused by the fact that the 0-degree imaging plane transects the posterior leaflet near the junction of the anterolateral (P1) and middle (P2) scallop.

Table 1. Main mechanisms of Mitral Regurgitation by TEE

Etiology	TEE characteristics	Valve repair may require
Global LV dilatation (spherical instead of ellipsoid shape)	Annular dilatation Malapposition Malcoaptation Restricted motion Central jet	Annuloplasty

Degenerative MR	Annular dilatation
	Leaflet prolapse
	  malapposition and
	  normal coaptation
	Increased motion
	Eccentric jet
	  AMVL: posterior direction
	  PMVL: anterior direction
	Central jet
	
	  Prolapse AMVL and PMVL
	Flail leaflet
	malapposition and
	malcoaptation
		AMVL prolapse
		  Annuloplasty
		  Chordal shortening
		  Flip-over
		  Chordal transposition or
		  replacement
		PMVL prolapse
		  Annuloplasty
		  PMVL quadrangular
		  resection
		Chordal shortening
		Flail leaflet
		  Annuloplasty
		  Quadrangular resection
		  PMVL
		  Sliding valvuloplasty
		  Flip-over
		  Chordal transposition
		Commissural prolapse
		  Sliding valvuloplasty

Ischemic MR	Annular dilatation* Restricted motion Malapposition and normal coaptation by retraction of PMVL (scarring PM and/or posterolateral dyskinesia) Prolaps by PM elongation Flail leaflet by PM head rupture	Annuloplasty See above Reimplantation of ruptured PM

Endocarditis MR	Annular dilatation*
	Vegetation
	Leaflet perforation
	  regurgitation jet originating
	  outside the closure line
	  (f.e. at the leaflet base)
	Valve prolapse or flail leaflet
		Annuloplasty
		Debridement
		Leaflet patch or suture repair
		
		See above

Rheumatic MR	Annular dilatation Malapposition, malcoaptation, Restricted motion by thickened calcified leaflets and shortening of chordae and PM	Repair probably not feasible

Not always present

MR = Mitral Regurgitation; AMVL = anterior mitral leaflet; PMVL= posterior mitral leaflet; PM = papillary muscle

HOW TO ASSESS SEVERITY OF MITRAL REGURGITATION?

Semi-quantification of the severity of mitral regurgitation (MR) by TEE may be performed in several ways. Often various ways are combined to give an estimation of severity on a 4-point scale.

Assessment of the jet area

First the color gain is optimized so that the level is just below the point of appearance of "background" color noise artifacts in the image field. The sector angle is adjusted allowing visualization of the entire jet with a maximal possible frame rate. After that, the largest representation of the jet is searched throughout the entire 180^0 arch of imaging planes. The jet area is measured by tracing the turbulent jet area (mosaic appearance) and the adjoining layer of laminar flow away from the mitral valve. Jet area dimensions are influenced not only by the regurgitant volume or severity of mitral regurgitation. They are also affected by instrument settings (gain, pulse repetition frequency, transducer frequency and wall filter settings) and systolic driving pressure (i.e. the same regurgitant volume leads to a larger jet area if the driving pressure is higher). In addition, it is important to realize that eccentric jets (adhering to the atrial wall) have a higher regurgitant volume than central (free) jets of the same area[8]. Nevertheless, the severity of regurgitation obtained by intra-operative TEE seems to correlate well with early post-operative TTE and left ventricular angiographic severity[9].

Pieper et al.[10] using left ventricular angiography as a gold standard for severity of MR and monoplane TEE found that the optimal cut-off value for jet area indicating severe grade III or IV MR was lower in eccentric jets than in central jets (5 cm^2 vs. 8 cm^2). In anaesthetized patients, sensitivity, specificity, and positive and negative predictive value of jet area of ≥ 5 cm^2 for grade III or IV mitral regurgitation were 67%, 100%, 100%, and 50% respectively. Flaschkampf et al.[11] using left ventricular angiography as a gold standard for severity of MR and multiplane TEE, found an optimal cut-off value for jet area of 7.8 cm^2. They found no different optimal cut-off value of jet area for eccentric compared to central jets and noticed an important overlap of jet areas between angiographic grades.

Proximal jet diameter

The proximal jet diameter is measured in the image plane in which the minimal diameter of the jet, just after passing the leaflets (vena contracta), appears the largest. Several studies have reported a best cut-off value between grade I/II and grade III/IV MR of 0.6 to 0.65 cm.[4,12] Overestimation of regurgitation with this method may occur if the regurgitant orifice is slit like rather than circular.

Assessment of the size of the proximal convergence zone

Proximal to a regurgitant orifice one can recognize a red-blue aliasing radius of flow accelerating towards the regurgitant orifice. This proximal flow convergence zone is interrogated using a color flow imaging sector as small as possible to maximize frame rate and by "zooming" the image. The baseline of the color bar velocity is shifted toward the transducer thus lowering the aliasing velocity to maximize the radius from the regurgitant orifice to the first aliasing point. The largest proximal convergence zone with an approximately hemispherical appearance is used for measurements. From the proximal convergence zone the maximal instantaneous flow rate (Q) in ml/sec can be calculated as $Q_{max} = 2 \pi r^2 * V_{alias}$ where r = radius to first alias in cm and V = velocity in cm/sec. The regurgitant orifice area (ROA) in cm^2 may be calculated as $ROA = Q_{max} / V_{max}$, where V_{max} is the maximal velocity of the regurgitant jet in m/sec measured by continuous wave Doppler.

Flaschkampf et al.[11] found an optimal cut-off value indicating severe (grade III or IV) mitral regurgitation at a maximal instantaneous flow rate of 190 ml/sec and a regurgitant orifice area of 0.4 cm^2. It is important to always take care that the proximal flow convergence area has a hemispheric contour shape.

Overestimation of regurgitant flow may occur when an adjacent left ventricular wall constraints the proximal flow field.[13] In those eccentric convergence areas a correction may be applied by multiplying the regurgitant flow rate with $\alpha/180$, where α is the convergence angle.

Assessment of pulmonary venous flow

Pulmonary flow should be assessed in the left and right upper pulmonary vein. The left upper pulmonary vein which enters the left atrium just lateral to the left atrial appendage can be visualized starting with a mid esophageal 4 chamber view by withdrawing the probe slightly and turning it to the left. The right upper pulmonary vein is imaged by turning the probe to the right at the level of the left atrial appendage. The lower pulmonary veins are less suitable for Doppler examination of pulmonary flow as they run in a perpendicular direction to the Doppler beam.

Pulmonary venous flow is determined by placing the pulsed Doppler sample volume 1 to 2 cm inside the pulmonary vein. Normal pulmonary venous flow consists of three waves: the S wave during ventricular systole, the D wave during ventricular diastole and the AR wave representing flow reversal in the pulmonary veins when the atrium contracts. Normally the systolic velocity is higher than the diastolic velocity. Mitral regurgitation of increasing severity results in blunting and ultimately reversal of the S wave.[14,15,16] In other words the systolic-to-diastolic flow ratio normally is ≥ 1; in blunted systolic flow it is between 0 and 1. There may exist a discordant flow pattern between the left and right upper pulmonary vein in 24 to 37% of the patients. This discordant pattern is mainly found in eccentric jets with an anterior direction, where the left upper pulmonary vein may show a normal flow pattern whereas there is systolic flow reversal in the right pulmonary vein. If one uses pulmonary venous flow as a measure for severity of MR it has to be remembered that blunting of systolic flow also may be caused by atrial fibrillation or an elevated left atrial pressure (mean > 15 mmHg) by other causes[17].

Which method to use for assessment of severity of mitral regurgitation?
Flaschkampf et al.[1] compared the above mentioned 5 methods for detection of angiographic grade III and IV MR and found that maximal regurgitant flow rate, regurgitant orifice area and regurgitant jet diameter excluded severe regurgitation with an accuracy of 90 % or more; see table 2.

Table 2. Transesophageal echocardiographic methods for the detection of severe
Mitral Regurgitation (angiographic grade III and IV)

Regurgitant parameter	Cut-off value	Sensitivity	Specificity	PPV	NPV
Color jet area	7.8 cm^2	85	80	74	89
PVF ratio	- 0.1	70	90	82	82
Proximal jet diameter	0.65 cm	90	83	79	92
Q max	190 ml/sec	100	93	91	100
ROA	0.4 cm^2	100	93	91	100

PPV= positive predictive value; NPV= negative predictive value;
PVF= ratio of peak systolic to peak diastolic pulmonary venous flow velocity.
In systolic retrograde flow, peak systolic flow velocity was noted as an negative number;
Qmax= maximal regurgitant flow rate; ROA= regurgitant orifice area
Reprinted with permission from The Journal of the American Society of Echocardiography 1998;
11:882-92 Flaschskampf et al.

Surgical assessment of the severity of mitral regurgitation
Methods that may be applied by the surgeon to assess the severity of mitral regurgitation are less than ideal.
Searching for a palpable thrill may miss eccentric jets. Filling of the arrested ventricle with fluid and inspecting the atrial aspect of the mitral valve for leakage disregards the influence of left ventricular geometry during normal contraction.

DOES INTRAOPERATIVE TEE DURING MITRAL VALVE REPAIR PREDICT EARLY AND LATE MITRAL VALVE DYSFUNCTION?

The intraoperative echocardiographic study for assessment of the results of mitral valve repair should start after cardiopulmonary bypass has been discontinued and the hemodynamic situation of the patient has stabilized. The loading conditions should resemble as much as possible loading conditions as they would be in the ambulatory state and the intravascular volume should be repleted[9][11]. In order to obtain this situation often blood pressure has to be raised pharmacologically by phenylephrine and/or with volume expansion.

Pitfalls in intraoperative assessment of the results of mitral valve repair
Image quality postrepair may be impaired by a dried probe in the esophagus, non-aspirated air from the stomach, a small or empty left atrium, air bubbles within the left atrium, invagination of the left atrial appendage, trapped air in the posterior pericardium or spontaneous contrast interfering with the color Doppler signal[19].
Transient mitral regurgitation may occur in several conditions. Mihaileanu et al.[19] found transient mitral regurgitation in 12 of 62 (20%) of their patients. This was caused by temporary impairment of left ventricular function[5], volume depletion[2], left ventricular outflow obstruction exacerbated by isoproterenol and nitroglycerine and abnormal ventricular activation (ventricular ectopic rhythm in 2 and epicardial pacing in 2).

What severity of mitral regurgitation assessed by intraoperative tee will allow satisfactory late results?
In a case-control study from the Cleveland Clinic, short-term- and long-term outcomes were determined of 76 patients with a "less than echo-perfect" result postrepair[20]. These patients were compared with a group of 76 patients with an "echo-perfect result", matched for age, sex, concomitant cardiac surgery, and impaired left ventricular function. Residual mitral regurgitation (MR) was assessed with monoplane TEE using the spatial distribution of the maximal MR jet as a fraction of the left atrial area. A "less than echo-perfect" result was defined as an average percentage of the left atrium subtended by the mitral regurgitation jet of $\leq 35\%$. They found that patients with grade 1 or 2 MR on their postpump echocardiogram had a threefold increase in the annual reoperation rate for recurrent mitral valve dysfunction compared with the rate in patients with no or trivial MR post repair (6% vs. 2% per patient-year). Mortality and morbidity (thrombo-embolic events, hospitalizations for heart failure and functional class) were not significantly different between both groups. They could find no factors predictive of late failure of mitral repair and noted all except one of the previous sites of repair to be intact.
In 1991-1992 a multicenter study ("ESMIR" study) was performed in the Netherlands (8 centers) and Belgium (1 center). In this study 159 patients underwent mitral valve repair; 62% of them underwent concomitant cardiac procedures (40% coronary bypass surgery, 15% aortic valve replacement, 11% tricuspid valve reconstruction). Residual mitral regurgitation (MR) was assessed with monoplane TEE using the maximal MR jet area: jet area < 2 cm^2 was defined as grade 1 MR, 2 – 4 cm^2 as grade 2 MR and a jet area > 4 cm^2 as grade 3 MR. There was no residual mitral regurgitation after repair in 48% of patients (77/159), grade 1 residual MR in 28% (45/159), grade 2 MR in 18% (29/159) and grade 3 in 5% (8/159). A second pump run because of failed repair was necessary in 12% of patients. The risk of re-operation within 1 year post mitral valve repair in patients with residual MR postpump was 6 times higher than in patients without residual MR (8% vs. 1%; RR 6.51, 95%CI 1.08-39.3). In patients with or without residual MR postpump, mortality or the incidence of congestive heart failure within 1 year were not significantly different. After 5 – 6 years following mitral valve repair 102 of 157 (65%) of patients had residual MR and 16 of 157 (10%) had undergone a reoperation of the mitral valve (Personal communication, EPG Pieper; 2000).
In the literature grade 1 and 2 MR after mitral valve repair are generally considered acceptable, although definitions of grade 1 and 2 MR differ among studies.[20, 9] Some use

jet area, others the ratio of jet area to left atrial area. Other measures of severity have not been applied in medium term follow-up studies.

In some circumstances one might accept more residual MR, for example after aortic valve replacement, coronary bypass grafting, or in patients with severe left ventricular dysfunction or extensive calcification of the mitral annulus. Evidently, residual prolapse is unacceptable.

Complications after mitral valve repair
Systolic anterior motion (SAM)

Systolic anterior motion (SAM) has been reported in a study from the Mayo Clinic to occur in 9% of patients[21]. SAM occurs primarily in patients with degenerative mitral valve disease, in the presence of a small and hypercontractile left ventricle and almost exclusively after implantation of a ring in the mitral annulus (more often with a rigid than flexible ring). SAM of mitral leaflets is due not only to the Venturi effect, but also to an anterior shift of the coaptation point of the anterior and posterior mitral leaflet. Maslow et al[22]. , have demonstrated that a relatively greater contribution of the posterior leaflet to the coaptation of the mitral valve was uniformly found in patients who exhibited SAM after repair (anterior leaflet length / posterior leaflet length ratio $\leq$ 1.3 in the 0^0 transverse view). Another predictor for SAM post mitral valve repair in this study was a smaller distance of the coaptation point of the mitral valve to the interventricular septum (C – septum $\leq$ 2.5 cm in the 0^0 transverse view).

The initial management of SAM postrepair consists of correction of a possible volume deplete and hypercontractile condition of the left ventricle by volume expansion, discontinuation of positive inotropic medication, adding a β-blocker and/or increasing the afterload with phenylephrine.

If residual MR $\geq$ grade 3 persists than the mitral valve repair result should be revised aiming to shift the coaptation point of the mitral valve backward, for example by a sliding technique.

Impaired left ventricular function
Impaired left ventricular function. Air emboli or entrapment of the circumflex artery in suturing near the mitral annulus may cause regional left ventricular wall motion abnormalities and consequently mitral regurgitation.

Suture dehiscence
Suture dehiscence may occur leading to perforation of a valve leaflet or partial dehiscence of the annuloplasty ring.

Mitral stenosis
Mitral stenosis may occur, especially after repair of rheumatic mitral regurgitation or an Alfieri mitral repair. A mitral valve area of $\leq$ 1.5 cm^2 in a normal adult should not be accepted.

EVALUATION OF MITRAL PROSTHESES BY TRANSESOPHAGEAL ECHOCARDIOGRAPHY

Assessment of anatomic abnormalities

Because of the vicinity of the oesophagus to the left atrium and mitral valve, high quality images can be obtained of prosthetic valves in mitral position.

Abnormal echoes associated with prosthetic valves are spontaneous echo contrast (SEC), microbubbles or cavitations, strands, sutures, vegetations and thrombus. Ionescu et al. recently have provided definitions for these abnormal echoes[23]. Spontaneous echo contrast (SEC) is defined as smoke-like echoes with slow swirling motion and is caused by slow flow (for example because of a low cardiac output or severe left atrial dilatation). However, SEC may also indicate slow flow due to pathologic obstruction of a mitral prosthesis. The prevalence of SEC is 7 - 53%. Microbubbles (or cavitations) are characterized by a discontinuous stream of rounded strongly echogenic, fast moving, transient echoes occurring when there is motion of the occluder of the prosthetic valve. The prevalence of microcavitations is approximately 47%. Strands are continuous linear, thin, mildly echogenic, mobile echoes. They are often visible intermittently during the cardiac cycle but are recurring at the same site. Strands are found in 6 to 47% of patients and are probably composed of fibrin. Sutures are defined as linear, thick, bright, multiple, evenly spaced, usually immobile echoes consistently seen at the periphery of the sewing ring of a prosthetic valve; they may be mobile when loose or unusually long. Vegetations and thrombus can not be distinguished by echocardiography alone; the differential diagnosis of these sessile or pedunculated masses depends on the full clinical picture. They may be interpreted as vegetations in a febrile patient and as thrombus in a poorly anticoagulated patient.

Prosthetic valve integrity and motion can be evaluated accurately with TEE. For bioprostheses evidence of leaflet degeneration (leaflet thickening, calcification or tear) can be identified. In mechanical valves abnormal disc excursion or a stuck leaflet can be visualized. Prosthetic valve dehiscence is characterized by a rocking motion of the entire prosthesis. An annular abscess may be recognized as an echo lucent, irregularly shaped area adjacent to the sewing ring of the prosthetic valve. Sometimes an abscess is echo dense.

Prosthetic valve obstruction

All normally functioning mechanical prosthetic valves show some obstruction to forward flow. Obstruction to flow may be determined by TEE by measuring the mean gradient and pressure half time. With the interpretation of the mean gradient one should realize that the mean gradient is not only dependent on the orifice area. Mean gradient also depends on heart rate (the faster the heart rate, the shorter the duration of diastole and the higher the transprosthetic gradient) and on transprosthetic stroke volume (higher in paravalvular leakage). The effective orifice area using the continuity equation can best be determined by transthoracic echocardiography (TTE). Pressure half time (P½ - time) as a measure of obstruction should also be interpreted with great caution. It is not only determined by orifice area but also by the early diastolic transprosthetic pressure gradient, heart rate and compliance of left atrium and left ventricle. In general practice, in a symptomatic patient with a mitral prosthesis and a heart rate of 70 – 100 per minute, pathologic obstruction of the valve prosthesis might be suspected if the mean pressure gradient is > 10 mm Hg and the P½ - time > 160 msec. It is important however, to interpret the aforementioned values of mean gradient and P½ - time in the clinical context of the patient and to look for morphologic abnormalities of the prosthetic valve. Pathologic valve obstruction may be caused by valve thrombosis, tissue in growth and sometimes by a vegetation interfering with normal disc motion.

Acute immobilization of a mechanical prosthesis disc (so called sticking disc) is a rare but life-threatening complication often caused by chord remnants or stitches. This can be easily visualized by TEE.

A high transprosthetic gradient despite a normally functioning prosthetic valve may occur after implantation of a valve prosthesis that is too small for the patient's body surface area (Valve Prosthesis – Patient mismatch). This is discussed in another chapter.

Prosthetic valve leakage

Prosthetic valves can be divided in mechanical and bioprosthetic valves. In vitro studies have demonstrated that mechanical prosthesis have closure backflow (necessary to close the valve) and leakage backflow (starting after valve closure).

The closure and leakage backflow pattern is dependent on the prosthesis design. For example tilting disc valves (like St. Jude Medical and Medtronic Hall valves) do not rest on a ledge of the orifice ring but fit inside the ring with a small space between the disc and ring or disc and pivot. Leakage backflow occurs through these small spaces, and generates specific jet patterns within the left atrium. Ball-in-cage prostheses however consist of a poppet, which rests on the ledge once the valve has been closed leaving no space between ring and ball. Therefore, Starr Edwards valves show only closure backflow and no leakage backflow. See table 3.

Table 3. Normal patterns of back flow in prosthetic valves[24]

	Duration	Central jets	Peripheral jets	Backflow Volume (cc per cycle)
Mechanical prostheses				
Starr Edwards	Early systole	0	2, confluent	4
Björk Shiley	Holosystolic	0	2	8
Medtronic Hall	Holosystolic		2	5.5
	Mid + late Systolic	1		
St.Jude Medical	Holosystolic	1-2	2	4.5
Bioprostheses				
Stented	Early	1	0	2
Stentless	Early	1	0	
Homografts		0	0	

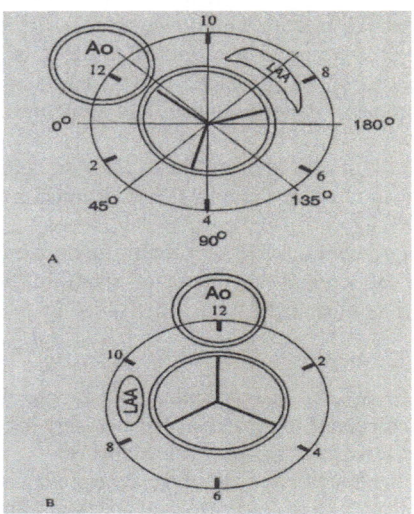

Figure 2. *Reference view displaying the prosthetic mitral valve and its relationship to the aortic root (Ao) and left atrial appendage (LAA) as seen from the left ventricular apex. The hours of a clock face corresponding to those shown in the surgical perspective, have been overlaid.*
(B) Surgical view of prosthetic mitral valve and its relationship to the aortic root.
Reprinted with permission from the Society of Thoracic Surgeons. (The Annals of Thoracic Surgery 1998; 65: 1025-31) Foster GP et al.

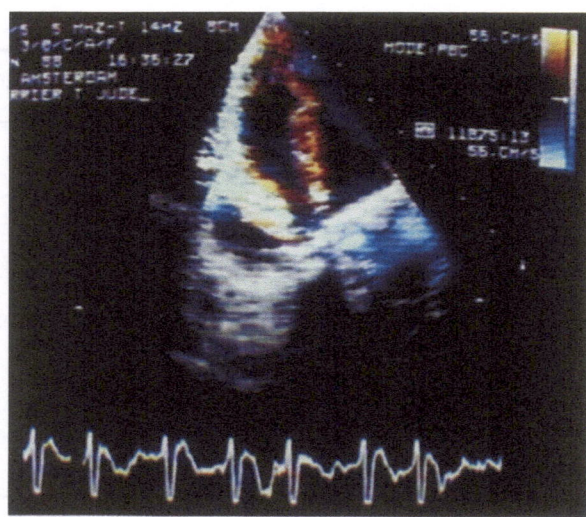

Figure 3. Normal backflow low-velocity nonaliasing jet encoded in a homogeneous colour and pathologic turbulent crescent shaped jet adhering to the left atrial wall.
(Reprinted with permission from American Journal of Cardiology; 1989; 63:1471-4 van den Brink et a)l.

Pathologic regurgitation is divided in paravalvular and valvular regurgitation. Evaluation of a prosthetic valve for regurgitation is done by centrring the prosthetic valve in the midesophageal four-chamber view. Then the sewing ring is imaged in full by rotation of the imaging plane from 0 ^{0} to 180 ^{0}, keeping the sewing ring in the centre of the image, making small adjustments of the transducer tip. See figure 2. Anatomic landmarks for localization of paravalvular leakage and for communication with the surgeon are the aorta and left atrial appendage. Pathologic regurgitation can be distinguished from normal backflow by the Color Doppler appearance of the jets. See figure 3. Normal closure and leakage backflow jets are low-velocity nonaliasing jets encoded in a homogeneous color (red in mitral valve prostheses). In contrast, pathologic jets are more turbulent and extensive, they are often eccentric (crescent shaped) and adherent to the left atrial wall. Pathologic regurgitation in mechanical valves may be caused by prosthetic valve dehiscence or by interference of structures (f.e. thrombus or vegetations) with disc closure. In bioprosthetic valves pathologic regurgitation may be caused by prosthesis dehiscence or leaflet degeneration (calcification or tear).

Severity of pathologic regurgitation is assessed by measurement of jet area, assessment of the pulmonary vein flow (looking for systolic flow reversal), and determination of diastolic forward transprosthetic flow (increased mean gradient and short P ½ time). Jet area measurement in eccentric jets may underestimate the severity of regurgitation because of the Coanda effect (spreading of the jet along the atrial wall).

CONCLUSION

Transesophageal two-dimensional and Doppler echocardiography is a valuable tool for the evaluation of mitral prosthesis dysfunction and the intraoperative assessment of the result of mitral valve repair. It provides unique information on both anatomy and function of the mitral valve in the beating heart. Mechanism and severity of mitral regurgitation can be determined. However, for successful application of transesophageal echocardiography both surgeons and echocardiographers should have a thorough knowledge of possibilities and limitations of the technique and they should "understand each others language". More studies are needed that evaluate short and long-term results of mitral valve repair in relation to postpump MR severity using the size of the proximal convergence zone and width of the vena contracta of the residual MR rather than jet area.

Three-dimensional echocardiography for assessment of the mechanism of mitral regurgitation is a promising technique but still has not found wide application in clinical practice because it remains time consuming and is not able to give "on-line" information.

42

REFERENCES

1. Enriquez-Sarano M, Schaff HV, Orszulak TA, Tajik AJ, Baily KR, Frye RL. Valve repair improves the outcome of surgery for mitral regurgitation. A multivariate analysis. Circulation 1995; 91: 1022-28.

2. ASE/SCA guidelines for performing a comprehensive intraoperative multiplane transesophageal echocardiography examination: recommendations of the American Society of Echocardiography council for intraoperative echocardiography and the society of cardiovascular anesthesiologists task force for certification in perioperative transesophageal echocardiography. J Am Soc Echocardiogr 1999; 12: 884-900.

3. Pieper EP, Hellemans IM, Hamer HP, Ravelli AC, van den Brink RBA, Ebels T, Lie KI, Visser CA. Additional value of biplane transesophageal echocardiography in assessing the genesis of mitral regurgitation and the feasibility of valve repair. Am J Cardiol 1995; 75: 489-93.

4. Pepi M, Barbier P, Doria E, Bortone F, Tamborini G. Intraoperative multiplane vs. biplane transesophageal echocardiography for the assessment of cardiac surgery. Chest 1996; 109: 305-11.

5. Hellemans IM, Pieper EG, Ravelli ACJ, Hamer JPM, Jaarsma W, Van den Brink RBA, Peels CH, van Swieten HA, Tijssen JGP, Visser CA, on behalf of the ESMIR research group. Comparison of transthoracic and transesophageal echocardiography with surgical findings in mitral regurgitation. Am J Cardiol 1996; 77: 728-33.

6. Stewart WJ, Currie PJ, Salcedo EE, Klein AL, Marwick T, Agler DA, Homa D, Cosgrove DM. Evaluation of mitral leaflet motion by echocardiography and jet direction by Dopplercolor flow mapping to determine the mechanism of mitral regurgitation. J Am Coll Cardiol 1992; 20: 1353-61.

7. Grewal KS, Malkowski MJ, Kramer CM, Dianzumba S, Reichek N. Multiplane transesophageal echocardiographic identification of the involved scallop in patients with flail mitral valve leaflet: intraoperative correlation. J Am Soc Echo 1998; 11: 966-71

8. Enriquez-Sarano M, Tajik AJ, Bailey KR, Seward JB. Color flow imaging compared with quantitative Doppler assessment of severity of mitral regurgitation: influence of eccentricity of jet and mechanism of regurgitation. J Am Coll Cardiol 1993; 21: 1211-19.

9. Reichert SLA, Visser CA, Moulijn AC, Suttorp MJ, van den Brink RBA, Koolen JJ, Jaarsma W, Vermeulen F, Dunning AJ. Intraoperative transesophageal color-coded Doppler echocardiography for evaluation of residual regurgitation after mitral valve repair. J Thorac Cardiovasc Surg 1990; 100: 756-61.

10. Pieper EPG, Hellemans IM, Hamer HPM, Ravelli ACJ, Cheriex EC, Tijssen JGP, Lie KI, Visser CA. Value of systolic pulmonary venous flow reversal and color Doppler jet measurements assessed with transesophageal echocardiography in recognizing severe pure mitral regurgitation. Am J. Cardiol. 1996; 78: 444-50.

11. Flachskampf FA, Frieske R, Engelhard B, Grenner H, Frielingsdorf J, Beck F, Reineke T, Thomas JD, Hanrath P. Comparison of transesophageal Doppler methods with angiography for evaluation of the severity of mitral regurgitation. J Am Soc Echocardiogr 1998; 11: 882-92.

12. Grayburn PA, Fehske W, Omran H, Brickner ME, Lüderitz B. Multiplane transesophageal echocardiographic assessment of mitral regurgitation by Doppler color flow mapping of the vena contracta. Am J Cardiol 1994; 74: 912-17.

13. Pu M, Vandervoort PM, Griffin BP, Leung DY, Stewart WJ, Cosgrove DM, Thomas JD. Quantification of mitral regurgitation by the proximal convergence method using tranesophageal echocardiography. Circulation 1995; 92: 2169-77.

14. Klein AL, Obarski TP, Stewart WJ, Casale PN, Pearce GL, Husbands K, Cosgrove DM, Salcedo EE. Transesophageal Doppler cehocardiography of pulmonary venous flow: a new marker of mitral regurgitation severity. J Am Coll Cardiol 1991; 18: 518-26.

15. Klein AL, Bailey AS, Cohen GI, Stewart WJ, Duffy CI, pearce GL, Slacedo EE. Importance of sampling both pulmonary veins in grading mitral regurgitation by transesophageal echocardiography. J Am Soc Echocardiogr 1993; 6: 115-23.
16. Kamp O, Huitink H, van Eenige MJ, Visser CA, Roos JP. Value of pulmonary venous flow characteristics in the assessment of severity of native mitral valve regurgitation: an angiographic correlated study. J Am Soc Echocardiogr 1992; 5: 239-46.
17. Kuecherer HF, Muhiudeen IA, Kusomoto FM.. Estimation of mean left atrial pressure from transesophageal pulsed Doppler echocardiography of pulmonary venous flow. Circulation 1990; 82: 1127-39.
18. Czer LSC, Maurer G, Bolger AF, De Robertis M, Resser KJ, Kass RM, Lee ME, Blanche C, Chaux A, Gray RJ, Matloff M. Left ventricular afterload: an important determinant of mitral regurgitant jet size by color Doppler flow mapping. Circulation 1987; 76 [Suppl IV]: IV-449
19. Mihaileanu S, El Asmar B, Acar A, Lamberti A, Diebold B, Perier P, Dreyfus G, Bensasson D, Dang Y, Iliesu D, CarpentierA. Intra-operative transoesophageal echocardiography after mitral valve repair-specific conditions and pitfalls. Eur Heart J 1991; 12 (Suppl. B):26-9.
20. Fix J, Isada L, Cosgrove D, miller DP, Savage R, Blum J, Stewart W. Do patients with less than echo-perfect results from mitral valve repair by intraoperative echocardiography have a different outcome? Circulation 1993; 88 [part 2]: 39-48.
21. Freeman WK, Schaff HV, Khandheria BK, Oh JK, Orszulak TA, Abel MD, Seward JB, Tajik AJ. Intraoperative evaluation of mitral valve regurgitation and repair by transesophageal echocardiography: incidence and significance of systolic anterior motion. J Am Coll Cardiol 1992; 20: 599-609.
22. Maslow AD, Regan MM, Haering JM, Johnson RG, Levine RA. Echocardiographic predictors of left ventricular outflow tract obstruction and systolic anterior motion of the mitral valve after mitral valve reconstruction for myxomatous valve disease. J Am Coll Cardiol 1999; 34: 2096-2104.
23. Ionescu AA, Moreno de la Santa P, Dunstan FD, Butchart EG, Fraser AG. Mobile echoes on prosthetic valves are not reproducible. Results and clinical implications of a multicenter study. Eur Heart J 1999; 20: 140-7.

LONG-TERM RESULTS OF PROSTHETIC DEVICES IN MITRAL POSITION

Dr. G.L. RIJK-ZWIKKER, Dr. B.J. DELEMARRE, Prof.Dr. R.A.E. DION

INTRODUCTION

In the early nineties several publications described the long-term outcome after mitral valve replacement, resulting in survival curves of up to 15 years. Freedom from valve related complications were calculated for large patient cohorts and risk factors were identified. The mortality-rate of patients with valve prostheses, was approximately twice as high as expected in the general population, resulting in a death rate of 5% patient per year for patients with prosthetic mitral valves[1-27].

The majority of patients operated upon 10 to 15 years ago were in the New York Heart Association functional class III to IV, before surgery was considered. Surgical treatment for mitral valve disease has shifted from valve replacement to valve repair, based on better long-term survival after repair. This shift has taken place in the last decennium, influenced by the changing pattern of mitral valve disease in the western world from rheumatic disease to ischemic mitral valve incompetence. Nevertheless, a large number of patients who have received a prosthetic mitral valve are still alive, and are therefore exposed to all the sequelae of this intervention.

In order to place results of mitral valve replacement in a perspective, the natural history of mitral valve disease, and the influence of concomitant disease such as atrial fibrillation and its complications, should be compared with the natural history of prosthetic mitral valve disease and its complications.

The purpose of this review of the literature is to evaluate the causes of death of patients with prosthetic mitral valve disease, and to focus on factors determining survival before and after mitral valve replacement, which may be altered by medical treatment, or may benefit from surgical intervention.

THE NATURAL HISTORY OF MITRAL INCOMPETENCE

The natural history of mitral incompetence due to mitral valve prolapse in an asymptomatic patient shows that 10% of the patients develop symptoms leading to surgical correction each year. Ten year survival is reported to be between 35% and 57%, even in the absence of symptoms. Horstkotte found no patients surviving for more than 10 years in his patient cohort with symptomatic mitral incompetence[29]. Poor survival is to some extend due to a high incidence of sudden death presumably from ventricular arrhythmia's[39,40,41]. Surgery on patients with preoperative NYHA class I/II results in an improved early and late survival both after valve repair and after valve replacement [33-38]. This is independent of left ventricular function and age.

ROLE OF ATRIAL FIBRILLATION

In sinus rhythm closure of the native mitral and tricuspid valve is induced by the spatial flow pattern within the ventricle. However, in the presence of atrial fibrillation, the valves closes as a result of pressure cross-over between ventricles and atria. Hence, in atrial fibrillation mitral valve incompetence and tricuspid incompetence are frequently encountered. The development of AF is associated with significantly lower CO, increased pulmonary artery pressure, wedge pressure, pulmonary resistance and increased right atrial pressure[31].

In addition, patients with a valve prosthesis and preoperative atrial fibrillation show lower long-term survival when compared with patients in sinus rhythm[9].

PRE-OPERATIVE DETERMINANTS FOR LATE SURVIVAL

Ling followed patients with a flail leaflet who had been treated medically, and found survival less than predicted. This was determined by age, presence of symptoms and ejection fraction. Surgery improved survival [34,35,36].

According to Tribouilly et al, one of the important preoperative risk factors for diminished survival in organic mitral regurgitation is pre-operative NYHA class III or IV [33]. This was evident both for valve repair and valve replacement. Reduced EF and concomitant CAD showed a similar pattern of decreased survival rate once patients became symptomatic. No correlation existed for ischemic mitral incompetence and mitral stenosis [33,36].

Rosen showed that the annual risk point for symptoms leading to surgery was 10.3% in a similar patient group with asymptomatic mitral incompetence. The change in RV ejection fraction during exercise predicted the likelihood of progression to symptoms [38].

Thus, late survival after mitral valve replacement is determined by the timing of the operation. In the absence of symptoms and atrial fibrillation, post-operative morbidity and mortality are significantly less, resulting in better long-term survival.

POSTOPERATIVE DETERMINANTS FOR LATE SURVIVAL AFTER MITRAL VALVE REPLACEMENT

The effect of specific surgical techniques with respect to preservation of part of the subvalvular apparatus has not been incorporated into many of the publications on long-term survival. Rheumatic heart disease means by definition that in the majority of the cases, the severely abnormal subvalvular apparatus has been resected at the time of surgery. Resection of the chordal apparatus has a known negative influence on left ventricular function [45-49]. If we regard the improved survival rate of mitral valve repair over replacement, as the difference in survival with and without subvalvular apparatus, it is obvious that the presence of the subvalvular apparatus is important for left ventricular function[33]. David found a ten-year survival rate of 80% with preservation of the subvalvular apparatus versus 63% survival for patients without chordal preservation. This holds true particularly for patients with mitral incompetence [45,46].

Comparison of tissue valves with mechanical valves in the mitral position, showed little or no difference with respect to long-term survival, valve related mortality and morbidity [10,11,22,26,43]. The Ionesco-Shiley pericardial valve and Bjork-Shiley mechanical valve are of course exceptions.

The subject of orientation of the valve prosthesis within the mitral annulus has been given little attention [50]. We have consequently not found any papers on the influence of valve orientation upon long-term survival.

The most common cause of death after mitral valve replacement is cardiac, non- valve related death. Causes of mortality and morbidity after mitral valve replacement are left and right ventricular failure, and sudden death [30,39,40,43]. Reoperations have a relatively high mortality rate. Structural valve deterioration of tissue valves is the most frequent indication for reoperation. Furthermore mortality and morbidity is related to thromboembolic- and bleeding complications. However, one cannot ignore data indicating that the presence of atrial fibrillation, decreased left ventricular function, coronary artery disease and advanced age before valve replacement, not only have a negative influence on early mortality, but also on late mortality and morbidity [32,33,44]. Five years after valve implantation, annual mortality rate is 4.6%. The mortality is lowest (2.8%) between one and five years after valve replacement [52,55,57].

Neurological complications may be major or fatal after embolic events or bleeding. In addition, recent publications suggest that high intensity signals (HITS), generated by all mechanical valves cause a chronic persistent flow of (gaseous) micro-emboli. It is suggested by Deklunder and currently also under investigation in our group, that the chronic persistent HITS may have a negative effect on cognitive functioning [51].

POST-OPERATIVE THROMBO-EMBOLIC EVENTS AND BLEEDING

Thromboembolic events and bleeding are classified as non-cardiac, valve related events. Risk factors for thromboembolic events are mitral valve prosthesis, atrial fibrillation, enlarged left atrium, low left ventricular ejection fraction, history of prior thromboembolic events. Additionally coronary artery disease and the presence of a pacemaker increases the risk for thrombo embolic events up to four times [52,55].

The incidence of thromboembolic events is reported to be between 0.9 and 2.1% per year for prosthetic mitral valves, after the initial three postoperative months have been passed. According to Cannegieter age is a significant factor [52,57]. Atrial fibrillation without mitral valve disease is a major source of thromboembolic events and thus should be treated with oral anticoagulants. Stein suggests addition of low dose aspirin for patients with coronary artery disease and stroke [54]. However, investigators from Leiden found in a meta-analysis no benefit from adding platelet inhibitors to coumadin therapy [52]. However Cappelleri using more recent cohorts in a meta-analysis, did indeed find some evidence that the incidence of stroke in patients with valve prosthesis, is lower if aspirin is added to the anticoagulation regimen, albeit at the expense of increased gastro-intestinal bleeding [55].

Bleeding invariably occurs as a complication of too high levels of anticoagulation. Van der Meer reports 42% more major bleeding complications for every one-point increase in INR. The incidence from major bleeding complications given in the literature varies between 1.6% and 5.2 % increasing with age [52,56]. Mortality from major bleeding ranks second as the cause of death in Horstkotte's publication on mitral stenosis and valve replacement [29]. In general, consensus exists that the "best" anticoagulation level of the first generation mitral valve prosthesis in the presence of atrial fibrillation (Starr Edwards Ball valve, Bork-Shiley Disk valves and MedtronicHall) is between INR 3,5 and 4.5. The bi-leaflet valves in the mitral position in patients with sinus rhythm without prior embolus carry a low risk at INR levels of 2.0 to 2.5 [52,56,57].

RE-OPERATIONS

The indications for reoperation may be classified as cardiac and valve related. The main indication for re-operation of mitral valve prostheses is structural deterioration of (tissue) valves, endocarditis, para- valvular defects, valve thrombosis, pannus formation and residual or recurrent tricuspid incompetence. Depending on the age of the patient the indication for re-operation may also be progressive coronary artery disease [58-66].

Risk factors for early mortality after reoperation are emergency operation for thrombosis of a prosthesis, acute endocarditis, acute valvular dehiscence with clinical deterioration, and surgical problems. Older age and NYHA class also play a major role [61,63]. Risk factors for late mortality after re-reoperation are recurrent para-valvular dehiscence, with or without endocarditis and tricuspid incompetence. In recent years peri-operative mortality has decreased substantially and elective surgical procedures show a similar peri-operative mortality to the initial operation [63,64,65].

Single mitral valve re-replacement on an elective basis in a patient with a normal left and right ventricular function is reported to carry a low risk of 1.5 % [58,65]. The peri-operative mortality increases with emergency operation up to 40%, double valve replacement to 22%, with poorer NYHA class, (from 2.2% to 15.5%), concomitant procedures to 16 % [66]. Not surprisingly the 5 and 10 year survival after re-replacement of the mitral valve is somewhat reduced, when compared to survival after the first valve replacement (78% and 37 to 52% respectively) [63,65,66].

ENDOCARDITIS

Endocarditis of mitral valve prostheses is an infection starting at the sewing ring of the prosthesis and extending into the peri-valvular tissue, resulting in tissue loss and dehiscence of the prosthesis. Endocarditis is also the major cause of para-valvular defects. The reported incidence of late endocarditis is between 2.5 and 3.7% [67-75]. The incidence is much higher (up to 20%) when valve replacement was performed because of previous endocarditis [71]. Ten-year survival is reported to be between 36% and 59% after valve replacement for endocarditis [70,71]. Initial treatment with the correct antibiotics is mandatory. Ongoing septicemia present for longer than 48 hours after the start of antibiotic treatment, and the presence of cerebral emboli are indications for surgical intervention, once cerebral bleeding is ruled out. However, once dehiscence is detected, hemodynamic deterioration is imminent and re-replacement should be performed immediately. Uncontrolled infection and abscess formation are also indications for urgent surgery. Tissue destruction is prominent in Staphylococcal aureus infections and carries a more serious prognosis [74,75]. The urgency of the procedure and the hemodynamic status of the patient determine peri-operative mortality. There is no consensus in the literature, as to whether mechanical valves or tissue valves differ in their susceptibility to endocarditis, or whether the type of valve used for the replacement changes outcome [63]. The complete excision of infected tissue is probably a more important factor in combating recurrence of infection, than the type of prosthesis used for replacement of the infected valve prosthesis.

POST-OPERATIVE PULMONARY HYPERTENSION

Pulmonary hypertension is persistent resistance after valve. Sometimes, the increased pulmonary pressure is only prominent during exercise [76]. This masked pulmonary hypertension may be the cause for right ventricular failure and secondary tricuspid incompetence, which is a major cause of death after mitral valve replacement [28,29,77,78]. Pulmonary pressure may also be elevated, or may increase when left ventricular function is poor or deteriorates. Cesnjevar concludes that intervention in patients with mitral valve replacement and pulmonary hypertension carries a higher (11%) peri-operative mortality rate. However late survival rate is similar to primary replacement [78]. They conclude that even in the presence of pulmonary hypertension the results of valve replacement are acceptable.
Surgical intervention should also be considered if a para valvular defect, with or without hemolysis, is the probable cause of right ventricular overload. The peri-operative mortality

is 6% in Genoni's series [79]. Structural valve deterioration of biological valves, in particular in those patients having received a tissue valve before the age of 60 years, should be kept in mind when the valve is in place for more than 10 years [3,4,6,7,80]. Lastly, if there is no direct explanation for a late increase in pulmonary pressure, for example more than 6 years after valve replacement with mechanical valve prosthesis, pannus formation on the prosthesis should be considered. Pannus causes a concentric narrowing of the valve ostium which may result in entrapment of the valve leaflet, resulting in either severe mitral incompetence or valve thrombosis. The frequency of this complication is approximately 0.8% patients per year [63]. Replacement of the prosthesis is the only option.

STRUCTURAL FAILURE

The incidence of structural valve failure in mechanical valves is low. Intervention for replacement of a valve at risk is only justified if the combined risk of peri-operative mortality and increased incidence of thrombo-embolic events in the first year after valve replacement exceeds the risk of valve failure [59]. For example, the reason to advice against replacement of the Duromedics bi-leaflet valve selectively, when leaflet escape was reported, the relative risk for valve failure was calculated to be less than 0.047 % patients per year. In contrast the calculated risk for structural failure for a specific cohort of high risk Bjork-Shiley valves in the mitral position approached 12.5 % patients per year in the larger sizes. Hence elective replacement for the Bjork Shiley valve was recommended [81,82,83].

Structural deterioration of tissue valves is a major indication for re-operation of prosthetic valves and accounts for more than half of all re-operations. Structural failure is inversely related to the age of the patient at the time of implantation, also to the mitral position, female gender and type of prosthesis (3,84). Approximately 30 to 65 % of the tissue valves have been replaced after 10 years and 50 to 70% at 15 years [8,20,25].

In patients with tissue valves in the mitral position, actuarial freedom from structural valve deterioration at 10 years is reported by Burton to be between 78 and 94.3% for patients over 70 years [3,84]. Structural deterioration and subsequent replacement of the tissue valve does not appear to have a negative influence on overall survival when compared with mechanical valves. In a comparative study between mechanical valves and tissue valves by Hammermeister, the reoperation related morbidity and mortality of tissue valves appeared to weigh against the thrombo-embolic and anticoagulation related complications of mechanical valves and long-term survival is similar for both patient cohorts [41].

Structural deterioration accelerates after 7-10 years and patients with a tissue valve should be followed on a yearly basis, in order to prevent secondary right and left ventricular deterioration, as this increases the operative mortality.

PARAVALVULAR DEFECTS

In the literature the incidence of para-valvular leak after mitral valve replacement varies between 5% and 12.3%. It is lowest after mitral valve replacement for ischemic mitral disease (4.7%) and highest if the indication for valve replacement was endocarditis (up to 41.4%) or after a previous and recurrent para-valvular leak (35%) [41,43,79]. Poor tissue quality, (healed) endocarditis, extensive calcification of the annulus, and reoperation for valve degeneration with extensive fibrosis of the annulus are risk factors for para-valvular defects.

The introduction of cardioplegic myocardial protection improved exposure of the mitral annulus, although the incidence of para-valvular defects did not decline. Indications for surgery for para-valvular leaks are NYHA class III/IV symptoms, hemolysis and high lactate dehydrogenate levels. Even with a reported peri-operative mortality of 6% to 20 %, survival may be significantly better after re-fixation or replacement of the valve in comparison to medical treatment [41,79]. Tissue valves have a lower tendency for para-valvular defects, when compared to mechanical valves [87]. This is probably related to the larger sewing ring of bioprosthetic valves compared with that of the mechanical valves.

VALVE THROMBOSIS

Valve thrombosis is a relatively rare complication in the presence of coumadin treatment with an incidence of 1 % per patient year for all valve positions. The incidence of mitral valve thrombosis is about 5 times higher than in the aortic valve [54]. Mitral valve thrombosis is also linked to low cardiac output [52]. The incidence of valve thrombosis is lowest in the bi-leaflet valves, higher in the disk valves and high in the caged ball valves [52,53]. The incidence of valve thrombosis and of thromboembolic events is highest in the first year, in particular in the first 30 days after valve implantation and decreases thereafter as a result of tissue overgrowth of the sewing ring [52,53,57]. The major cause of valve thrombosis is inadequate anticoagulation for a prolonged period of time. The risk for valve thrombosis and thrombo-embolic events is very low when anticoagulation is discontinued for only a few days [52,88]. Preferred treatment of mitral valve thrombosis is valve surgery; thrombolysis can be used as a bailout procedure [60].

PANNUS

Pannus is fibrous tissue which slowly accumulates on the sewing ring of both mechanical and tissue valve prosthesis. It is part of the physiological in-growth of the sewing ring. However, after a period of 6 years or longer, the fibrous sheath may extend into the orifice of the valve and interfere with valve function. Overgrowth is particularly present on the ventricular site in tilting disk valves [60]. In bi-leaflet valves the pannus formation is present at or near the hinges of the valves. Ultimately pannus may reduce the excursion of the disk and precipitate valve thrombosis. Because of the location of the pannus on top of the valve ring, echocardiographic detection is difficult, due to the dense echo of the titanium housing. One of the symptoms may be unexplained pulmonary hypertension in the presence of normal valve function, and normal left ventricular function. Also valve thrombosis with adequate INR levels may indicate mechanical obstruction of the valve. Treatment of pannus formation consists of replacement of the valve prosthesis.

SUMMARY

A ten-year survival rate for patients with mitral incompetence without surgical treatment is approximately 57%. Annual mortality rate is of over 6% per year. Survival for patients with mitral stenosis without surgery has a similarly poor prognosis. Patients with a mitral valve prosthesis survive better but still have half of the life expectancy of the general population. Long-term results of tissue valves and mechanical valves are similar with respect to survival. Pre-operative left ventricular function and the presence of atrial fibrillation determines survival. Postoperative factors are the incidence of endocarditis, para-valvular defects, major thrombo-embolic events and the need for emergency reoperation.
Age at implantation, female gender and NYHA class stratify the risks for death in tissue valves, while para-valvular defects with or without endocarditis are the primary cause for reoperation in mechanical valves. Cardiac death is based on deteriorating left ventricular function in mitral incompetence and failing right ventricular function in patients with mitral stenosis.

Table 1. 10 year survival and incidence of complications % per patient year

	MS	MI	Mech. V	Tissue V
Valve thrombosis	NA	NA	0.2	0
Thrombo-embolic events	4.7	1.9	1.09-2.3	0.4 – 2
Hemorrhage	2-4	0.4	0.57-2.7	0.36-0.9
Endocarditis	1.5	0.11	0.54	1.0
Structural deterioration	NA	NA	<0.047	>5
Para-valvular defects	NA	NA	0.19-0.31	0.3
Left ventricular failure (Sudden death)	5.7	4.3-8.2	NA	NA
Right ventricular failure	0.34			
Actuarial survival	20	38-57	43.1±1.5	50±2
Sudden death	5.7	6.3	0.5	
Reoperation	NA	NA	0.15	0.03-0.70

REFERENCES

1. Zellner JL, Kratz JM, Crumbley AJ 3rd, Stroud MR, Bradley SM, Sade RM, Crawford FA Jr. ((1999). Long-term experience with the St. Jude Medical valve prosthesis. Ann. Thorac.Surg 68; 1210-1218.

2. Baudet EM, Puel V, McBride JT, Grimaud JP, Roques F, Clerc F, Roques X, Laborde N. 1995 Long-term results of valve replacement with the St. Jude Medical prosthesis. J Thorac Cardiovasc Surg 109(5): 858-70.

3. Burdon TA, Miller DC, Oyer PE, Mitchell RS, Stinson EB, Starnes VA, Shumway NE 1992 Durability of porcine valves at fifteen years in a representative North American patient population. J Thorac Cardiovasc Surg 103 (2):238-51; discussion 251-2.

4. Cohn LH, Couper GS, Aranki SF, Kinchla NM, Collins JJ Jr 1991. The long-term follow-up of the Hancock Modified Orifice porcine bioprosthetic valve. J Card Surg 1991 Dec;6(4 Suppl):557-61.

5. Cohn LH, Couper GS, Aranki SF, Rizzo RJ, Adams DH, Collins JJ Jr 1994 The long-term results of mitral valve reconstruction for the "floppy" valve. J Card Surg 9 (2 Suppl): 278-81.

6. Jamieson WR, Burr LH, Munro AI, Miyagishima RT. 1998 Carpentier-Edwards standard porcine bioprosthesis: a 21-year experience Ann Thorac Surg. 66(6 Suppl):S40-3.

7. Jamieson WR, Ling H, Burr LH, Fradet GJ, Miyagishima RT, Janusz MT, Lichtenstein SV. 1998 Carpentier-Edwards supra-annular porcine bioprosthesis evaluation over 15 years. Ann Thorac Surg 66(6 Suppl):S49-52.

8. Jamieson WR. Modern cardiac valve devices: bioprostheses and mechanical prostheses: state of the art. 1993 J Card Surg 8 (1): 89-98.

9. Bessell JR, Gower G, Craddock DR, Stubberfield J, Maddern GJ. (1996). Thirty years experience with heart valve surgery: isolated mitral valve replacement. Aust N Z J Surg. 66(12):806-12.

10. Kawachi Y, Tokunaga K. 1990 Clinical comparative study between mitral mechanical and bioprosthetic valves--what is the benefit of bioprosthetic valves in the mitral position? Jpn Circ J. 54(12):1525-34.

11. Fradet GJ, Jamieson WR, Abel JG, Lichtenstein SV, Miyagishima RT, Ling H,Tyers GF. 1995 Clinical performance of biological and mechanical prostheses. Ann Thorac Surg. 60(2 Suppl):S453-8.

12. Jamieson WR, Miyagishima RT, Grunkemeier GL, Germann E, Henderson C, Fradet GJ, Burr LH, Lichtenstein SV (1999) Bileaflet mechanical prostheses performance in mitral position. Eur J Cardiothorac Surg 15(6): 786-94.

13. Myken P, Bech-Hanssen O, Phipps B, Caidahl K (2000) Fifteen years follow up with the St. Jude Medical Biocor porcine bioprosthesis. J Heart Valve Dis 9(3):415-22.

14. Actis Dato GM, Caimmi P, Aidala E, Bardi G, Trichiolo S, Flocco R, Trimboli S, Di Summa M, Poletti G (1999) Bovine pericardial bioprosthesis in mitral position. A ten-year follow-up. Minerva Cardioangiol 47(9): 275-83.

15. Podesser BK, Khuenl-Brady G, Eigenbauer E, Roedler S, Schmiedberger A, Wolner E, Moritz A. (1998) Long-term results of heart valve replacement with the Edwards Duromedics bileaflet prosthesis: a prospective ten-year clinical follow-up. J Thorac Cardiovasc Surg 115(5):1121-29.

16. Craver J. (1999) CarboMedics Prosthetic Heart Valve. Europ.J Cardio-Thor Surg. 15 Suppl 1 S3-S11.

17. Legarra JJ, Llorens R, Catalan M, Segura I, Trenor AM, de Buruaga JS, Rabago G, Sarralde A. Eighteen-year Follow-up after Hancock II Bioprosthesis Insertion. (1999) H Heart Valve Dis 8 : 16-24.

54

18. Torrregrosa S, Gomez-Plana J, Valera FJ, Caffarena J, Maronas JM, Garcia-Sanchez F, Peris J, Frias R, Caffarera JM. (1999) Long-term Clinical Experience with the Omnicarbon Prosthetic Valve. Ann Thor. Surg 68: 881-886.

19. Kawachi Y, Tanaka J, Tominaga R, Kinoshita K, Tokunaga K. (1992) More than ten years follow-up of the Hancock porcine Bioprosthesis in Japan. J of Thor.Cardio-vasc. Surg. 104:5-13

20. Nitter-Hauge S, Abdelnoor M, Svennevig JL (1996). Fifteen-year experience with the Medtronic-Hall valve prosthesis. A follow-up study of 1104 consecutive patients. Circulation 94(9 Suppl)II 105-8

21. Schwarz F, Bootger J, Ruffmann K, Scheurlen H, Olschewski M, Storch HH, Saggau W, Kubler W, (1986). Determinanten der langzeitprognose nach prothetischen Mitralklappen ersatz. Z f Kardiol 75: 646-649.

22. Yong-In Kim, Lasaffre E, Scheys I, Stalpeart G, Flaming W, Daenen,WJ. (1994) The Monostrut versus the MedtronicHall prosthesis: A prospective Randomized Study. H Heart valve Dis. 3,3: 254-259.

23. Caimmi PP, Di Summa M, Galloni M, Gastaldi L, Papillo B, Actis Dato GM, Agaccio G, Donegani E, Poletti G, Morea M (1998) Twelve-year follow up with the Sorin Pericarbon bioprosthesis in the mitral position. J Heart Valve Dis 1998 Jul;7(4):400-6

24. Renzulli A, Ismeno G, Bellitti R, Casale D, Festa M, Nappi GA, Cotrufo M (1997) Long-term results of heart valve replacement with bileaflet prostheses. J Cardiovasc Surg (Torino) 3:241-7

25. Cohn LH, Couper GS, Aranki SF, Kinchla NM, Collins JJ Jr (1991). The long-term follow-up of the Hancock Modified Orifice porcine bioprosthetic valve. J Card Surg 6(4 Suppl):557-61

26. Fiore AC, Barner HB, Swartz MT, McBride LR, Labovitz AJ, Vaca KJ, St Vrain J, Grunkemeier GL, Kaiser GC (1997) Mitral valve replacement: randomized trial of St. Jude and Medtronic Hall prostheses. Ann Thorac Surg 3:707-12; discussion 712-3

27. Fann JI, Miller DC, Moore KA, Mitchell RS, Oyer PE, Stinson EB, Robbins RC, Reitz BA, Shumway NE (1996) Twenty-year clinical experience with porcine bioprostheses. Ann Thorac Surg 62(5): 1301-11; discussion 1311-2

28. Remadi JP, Bizouarn P, Baron O, Al Habash O, Despins P, Michaud JL, Duveau D (1998) Mitral valve replacement with the St. Jude Medical prosthesis: a 15-year follow-up. Ann Thorac Surg 66(3): 762-7

29. Horstkotte D, Niehues R, Strauer BE 1991 Pathomorphological aspects, aetiology and natural history of acquired mitral valve stenosis. Eur Heart J. 12 Suppl B: 55-60.

30. Horstkotte D 1992 Arrhythmias in the natural history of mitral stenosis. Acta Cardiol 1992;47(2):105-13

31. Moreyra AE, Wilson AC, Deac R, Suciu C, Kostis JB, Ortan F, Kovacs T, Mahalingham B. (1998) Factors associated with atrial fibrillation in patients with mitral stenosis: a cardiac catheterization study. Am Heart J135(1):138-45.

32. Detter C, Fischlein T, Feldmeier C, Nollert G, Reichenspurner H, Reichart B. 1999 Mitral commissurotomy, a technique outdated? Long-term follow-up over a period of 35 years. Ann Thorac Surg.68(6):2112-8.

33. Tribouilly CM, Enriquez-Sarano M, Schaff HV, Orszulak TA, Bailey KR, Tajik AJ, Frye RL (1999). Impact of preoperative symptoms on survival after surgical correction of organic mitral regurgitation: rationale for optimizing surgical indications. Circulation 26; 99(3): 400-5.

34. Ling LH, Enriquez-Sarano M, Seward JB, Tajik AJ, Schaff HV, Bailey KR, Frye RL. 1996 Clinical outcome of mitral regurgitation due to flail leaflet. N Engl J Med. 7;335(19):1417-23

35. Enriquez-Sarano M, Schaff HV, Orszulak TA, Tajik AJ, Bailey KR, Frye RL 1995 Valve repair improves the outcome of surgery for mitral regurgitation. A multivariate analysis. Circulation 1995 91(4):1022-8

36. Ling LH, Enriquez-Sarano M. Long-term outcomes of patients with flail mitral valve leaflets. Coron Artery Dis. 2000 ;11(1):3-9.

37. Gramaglia B, Imazio M, Checco L, Villani M, Morea M, Di Summa M, Bonamini R, Rosettani E, Mangiardi L.(1999) Mitral valve prolapse. Comparison between valvular repair and replacement in severe mitral regurgitation J Cardiovasc Surg (Torino) 40(1):93-96.

38. Rosen SE, Borer JS, Hochreiter C, Supino P, Roman MJ, Devereux RB, Kligfield, P, Bucek J. (1994) Natural history of the asymptomatic/minimally symptomatic patient with severe mitral regurgitation secondary to mitral valve prolapse and normal right and left ventricular performance. Am J Cardiol.15;74(4):374-80.

39. Grigioni F, Enriquez-Sarano M, Ling LH, Bailey KR, Seward JB, Tajik AJ, Frye FH. Sudden death in mitral regurgitation due to flail leaflet J Am Coll Cardiol. 1999 Dec;34(7):2078-85. RL

40. Alvarez L, Escudero C, Figuera D, Castillo-Olivares JL (1992). Late sudden cardiac death in the follow-up of patients having a heart valve prosthesis. J Thorac Cardiovasc Surg 104(2): 502-10.

41. Hammermeister KE, Sethi GK, Henderson WG, Oprian C, Kim T, Rahimtoola S 1993 A comparison of outcomes in men 11 years after heart-valve replacement with a mechanical valve or bioprosthesis. Veterans Affairs Cooperative Study onValvular Heart Disease. N Engl J Med 6;328(18):1289-96

42. Cannegieter SC, Rosendaal FR, Wintzen AR, van der Meer FJ, Vandenbroucke JP,Briet E. 1995 Optimal oral anticoagulant therapy in patients with mechanical heart valves. N Engl J Med. 333(1):11-7.

43. Hwang MH, Burchfiel CM, Sethi GK, Oprian C, Grover FL, Henderson WG, Hammermeister K. 1994 Comparison of the causes of late death following aortic and mitral valve replacement. VA Co-operative Study on Valvular Heart Disease. J Heart Valve Dis. 3(1):17-24.

44. David TE, Armstrong S, Sun Z. 1995 Left ventricular function after mitral valve surgery. J Heart Valve Dis. Oct;4 Suppl 2:S175-80.

45. Reardon MJ, David TE 1999 Mitral valve replacement with preservation of the subvalvular apparatus Curr Opin Cardiol 14(2):104-10

46. Horskotte D, Schulte HD, Bircks W, Strauer BE 1993 The effect of chordal preservation on late outcome after mitral valve replacement: a randomized study. J Heart Valve Dis 2(2):150-8

47. Lee EM, Shapiro LM, Wells FC (1996) Importance of subvalvular preservation and early operation in mitral valve surgery. Circulation 94(9): 2117-23

48. Van Rijk-Zwikker GL, Schipperheyn JJ: 1988 The effect of a rigid mitral ring on the function of the valve and the left ventricle. Circ 78 (suppl.4): 379,

49. Sintek CF, Pfeffer TA, Kochamba G, Fletcher A, Khonsari S. 1995 Preservation of normal left ventricular geometry during mitral valve replacement. J Heart Valve Dis. 4(5):471-5

50. Van Rijk-Zwikker GL, Delemarre BJ, Huysmans HA. (1996). The orientation of the bi-leaflet CarboMedics valve in the mitral position determines left ventricular spatial flow patterns. Eur J Cardio-thorac Surg 10, 513-520.

51. Deklunder G, Roussel M, Lecroart JL, Prat A, Gautier C.1998) Microemboli in cerebral circulation and alteration of cognitive abilities in patients with mechanical prosthetic heart valves. Stroke. 1998 Sep;29(9):1821-6.

52. Cannegieter SC, Rosendaal FR, Briet E: Thrombo-embolic and bleeding complications in patients with mechanical heart valve prosthesis. Circulation 1994; 89:635-641

53. Horstkotte D, Schulte H, Bircks W, Strauer B (1993) Unexpected findings concerning thromboembolic complications and anticoagulation after complete 10 year follow up of patients with St. Jude Medical prostheses. J Heart Valve Dis 2(3): 291-301

54. Stein PD, Alpert JS, Dalen JE, Horstkotte D, Turpie AG. 1998 Antithrombotic therapy in patients with mechanical and biological prosthetic heart valves. Chest. 1998 Nov;114(5 Suppl):602S-610S. Review

55. Cappelleri JC, Fiore LD, Brophy MT, Deykin D, Lau J. 1995 Efficacy and safety of combined anticoagulant and antiplatelet therapy versus anticoagulant mono therapy after mechanical heart-valve replacement: a meta analysis. Am Heart J.130(3 Pt 1):547-52.

56. Van der Meer FJ, Rosendaal FR, Vandenbroucke JP, Briet E. 1993 Bleeding complications in oral anticoagulant therapy. An analysis of riskfactors. Arch Intern Med. 153(13):1557-62.

57. Heras M, Chesebro JH, Fuster V, Penny WJ, Grill DE, Bailey KR, Danielson GK, Orszulak TA, Pluth JR, Puga FJ, et al. 1995. High risk of thromboemboli early after bioprosthetic cardiac valve replacement. J Am Coll Cardiol 25(5):1111-9.

58. Yamak B, Ozsoyler, Ulus AT, Kiziltepe U, Katircioglu SF, Tasdemir O.(1999) Comparison of reoperation findings of the Carpentier-Edwards (standard) bioprosthesis and the St Jude bioimplant (formerly Liotta) in the mitral position. Cardiovasc Surg 1999 Dec;7(7):730-4

59. Rizzoli G, Bottio T, De Perini L, Scalia D, Thiene G, Casarotto D (1998). Multivariate analysis of survival after malfunctioning biological and mechanical prosthesis replacement Ann Thorac Surg. 66(6 Suppl):S88-94

60. Rizzoli G, Guglielmi C, Toscano G, Pistorio V, Vendramin I, Bottio T, Thiene G, Casarotto D 1999 Reoperations for acute prosthetic thrombosis and pannus: an assessment of rates, relationship and risks Eur J Cardiothorac Surg 16(1):74-80

61. Turina J, Turina M. Left ventricular function and valvular reoperations. J Heart Valve Dis. 1995 Oct;4 Suppl 2:S223-8; discussion S228-9.

62. Jamieson WR, Marchand MA, Pelletier CL, Norton R, Pellerin M, Dubiel TW, Aupart MR, Daenen WJ, Holden MP, David TE, Ryba EA, Anderson WN Jr (1997) Structural valve deterioration in mitral replacement surgery: Comparison of Carpentier-Edwards supra-annular porcine and Perimount pericardial bioprostheses. J Thorac Cardiovasc Surg. 118(2): 297-304.

63. Jones EL, Weintraub WS, Craver JM, Guyton RA, Shen Y 1994 Interaction of age and coronary disease after valve replacement: Implications for valve selection. Ann Thorac Surg 58(2):378-84; discussion 384-5

64. Jamieson WR, Munro AI, Burr LH, Germann E, Miyagishima RT, Ling H I 1995 Influence of coronary artery bypass and age on clinical performance after aortic and mitral valve replacement with biological and mechanical prostheses. Circulation 1995 Nov 1;92(9 Suppl):II101-6

65. Gill IS, Masters RG, Pipe AL, Walley VM, Keon WJ Can J Cardiol 1999 Nov;15(11):1207-10 Determinants of hospital survival following reoperative single valve replacement.

66. Syracuse DC, Bowman FO Jr, Malm JR. 1979 Prosthetic valve reoperations. Factors influencing early and late survival. J Thorac Cardiovasc Surg. 77(3):346-54

67. Horstkotte D 2000 Endocarditis: epidemiology, diagnosis and treatment. Z Kardiol 89 Suppl 4:IV2-11

68. Horstkotte Prosthetic valve Endocarditis HorstkotteD, Bodnar E, (Eds) in Infective endocarditis ICR Publishers 1991;229-26

69. Edwards MB, Ratnatunga CP, Dore CJ, Taylor KM 1998 Thirty-day mortality and long-term survival following surgery for prosthetic endocarditis: a study from the UK heart valve registry. Eur J Cardiothorac Surg (2):156-64

70. Mullany CJ, Chua YL, Schaff HV, Steckelberg JM, Ilstrup DM, Orszulak TA, Danielson GK, Puga FJ. 1995 Early and late survival after surgical treatment of culture-positive active endocarditis. Mayo Clin Proc. 70(6):517-25

71. Alexiou C, Langley SM, Stafford H, Lowes JA, Livesey SA, Monro JL 2000 Surgery for active culture-positive endocarditis: determinants of early and late outcome. Ann Thorac Surg 69(5):1448-54

72. Choussat R, Thomas D, Isnard R, Michel PL, Iung B, Hanania G, Mathieu P, David M, du Roy de Chaumaray T, De Gevigney G, Le Breton H, Logeais Y, Pierre-Justin E, de Riberolles C, Morvan Y, Bischoff N. 1999. Perivalvular abscesses associated with endocarditis; clinical features and prognostic factors of overall survival in a series of 233 cases. Perivalvular Abscesses French Multicentre Study. Eur Heart J 20(3):232-41

57

73. Farina G, Vitale N, Piazza L, De Vivo F, de Luca L, Cotrufo J. Long-term results of surgery for prosthetic valve endocarditis. J Heart Valve Dis 3(2):165-71

74. Kuyvenhoven JP, van Rijk-Zwikker GL, Hermans J, Thompson J, Huysmans HA (1994) Prosthetic valve endocarditis: analysis of risk factors for mortality. Eur J Cardiothorac Surg (8):420-4

75. Roder BL, Wandall DA, Espersen F, Frimodt-Moller N, Skinhoj P, Rosdahl VT 1997 A study of 47 bacteriemic Staphylococcus aureus endocarditis cases: 23 with native valves treated surgically and 24 with prosthetic valves.

76. Nellessen U, Inselmann G, Ludwig J, Jahns R, Capell AJ, Eigel P. 2000 Rest and exercise hemodynamics before and after valve replacement--a combined Doppler/catheter study. Clin Cardiol. 23(1):32-8

77. Gamra H, Zhang HP, Allen JW, Lou FY, Ruiz CE. 1999 Factors determining normalization of pulmonary vascular resistance following successful balloon mitral valvotomy. Am J Cardiol.83(3):392-5.

78. Cesnjevar RA, Feyrer R, Walther F, Mahmoud FO, Lindemann Y, von der Emde J 1998 High-risk mitral valve replacement in severe pulmonary hypertension--30 years experience Eur J Cardiothorac Surg 1998 Apr;13(4):344-51; discussion 351-2

79. Genoni M, Franzen D, Vogt P, Seifert B, Jenni R, Kunzli A, Niederhauser U, Turina M (2000) Paravalvular leakage after mitral valve replacement: improved long-term survival with aggressive surgery? Eur J Cardiothorac Surg 17(1):14-9

80. Jamieson WR, Burr LH, Miyagishima RT, Fradet GJ, Janusz MT, Tyers FO, MacNab J, Chan F (1995) Structural deterioration in Carpentier-Edwards standard and supraannular porcine bioprostheses. Ann Thorac Surg 60(2 Suppl): S241-7

81. Lindblom D, Rodriquez L, Bjork VO : 1989. Mechanical Failure of the Bjork-Shiley valve; J Thoracic and Cardiovasc Surg; 97:95-97

82. Steyerberg EW, Kallewaard M, van der Graaf Y, van Herwerden LA, Habbema JD. (2000) Decision analyses for prophylactic replacement of the Bjork-Shiley convexo-concave heart valve: an evaluation of assumptions and estimates. Med Decis Making 2000 ;1:20-3

83. van der Graaf Y, de Waard F, van Herwerden LA, Defauw J (1992) Risk of strut fracture of Bjork-Shiley valves. Lancet 1; 339 (8788):257-61

84. Pupello DF, Bessone LN, Hiro SP, Lopez-Cuenca E, Glatterer MS Jr, Angell WW, Brock JC, Alkire MJ, Izzo EG, Sanabria G 1995 Bioprosthetic valve longevity in the elderly: an 18-year longitudinal study. Ann Thorac Surg 60(2 Suppl):S270-4; discussion S275

85. Remadi JP, Bizouarn P, Baron O, Al Habash O, Despins P, Michaud JL, Duveau D. 1998 Mitral valve replacement with the St. Jude Medical prosthesis: a 15-year follow-up.Ann Thorac Surg.66(3):762-7.

86. Van Rijk-Zwikker GL, Huysmans HA (1986). The incidence and localization of para-valvular leaks in combined aortic and mitral valve replacement. in: Proceedings international workshop on the management of multivalvular heart disease, Nitterhauge S., ed. 1986; 24 Oslo, Norway

87. Von Segesser LK, Enz R, Baur E, Laske A, Carrel T, Gallino A, Turina M 1990 Long-term performance in mitral bioprosthesis Schweiz.Med Wochenschr.120(30) 1098-101

88. Wijdicks EF, Schievink WI, Brown RD, Mullany CJ 1998 The dilemma of discontinuation of anticoagulation therapy for patients with intracranial hemorrhage and mechanical heart valves. Neurosurgery 42(4):769-73

89. Duran CM 1994 Tricuspid valve surgery revisited. J Card Surg 9(2 Suppl):242-7

90. Tager R, Skudicky D, Mueller U, Essop R, Hammond G, Sareli P. 1998 Long-term follow-up of rheumatic patients undergoing left-sided valve replacement with tricuspid annuloplasty--validity of preoperative echocardiographic criteria in the decision to perform tricuspid annuloplasty.Am J Cardiol. 81(8):1013-6.

58

91. Staab ME, Nishimura RA, Dearani JA. 1999 Isolated tricuspid valve surgery for severe tricuspid regurgitation following prior left heart valve surgery: analysis of outcome in 34 patients. J Heart Valve Dis. 8(5):567-74.

92. Pellegrini A, Colombo T, Donatelli F, Lanfranchi M, Quaini E, Russo C, Vitali E 1992 Evaluation and treatment of secondary tricuspid insufficiency Eur J Cardiothorac Surg 6(6):288-96

93. Porter A, Shapira Y,Wurzel M, Sulkes J, Vaturi M,Adler Y, Sahar G,Sagie A 1999 Tricuspid Regurgitation late after Mitral Valve Replacement: Clinical and Echocardiographic Evaluation. J Heart Valve Did 8:57-62.

POSTOPERATIVE EVALUATION AFTER MITRAL VALVE SURGERY

Dr. F.A. FLACHSKAMPF

INTRODUCTION

In the evaluation of mitral valve disease echocardiography plays an eminent role. It has become the gold standard for the assessment of severity in mitral stenosis. Selection of patients for interventional valvuloplasty relies mainly on the morphology of the valve as shown by echocardiography. In mitral regurgitation, echo and especially transesophageal echo can assess severity and mechanism of the mitral valve, as well as left ventricular function, and is crucial for selecting candidates for valve repair as opposed to valve replacement. However, the role of echo is also critical in the intra-operative and post-operative management of the patient with mitral valve disease[1]. This review focuses on the information obtained from echo early after coming off cardiopulmonary bypass in mitral valve surgery and later.

GENERAL CONSIDERATIONS: INDICATIONS FOR AND GOALS OF THE POSTOPERATIVE ECHO STUDY

Every patient should be studied by echo after mitral valve surgery. However, the use of *intraoperative* echo varies widely depending on local availability. Probably the technically demanding procedures of valve repair derive the greatest benefit from echo, which ideally should be performed at the earliest possible point in time, which is when the patient comes off the cardiopulmonary bypass, but before the chest is closed.

Since the routine surgical therapy for mitral valve stenosis now is valve replacement, there are only two operative procedures for mitral valve disease to consider:
a) Mitral valve repair and
b) Mitral valve replacement.

The postoperative evaluation by echo has to determine whether a proper function of the (repaired or replaced) valve was achieved, and if there are complications of surgery affecting other structures (Table 1).

POSTOPERATIVE EVALUATION OF MITRAL VALVE REPAIR

The most important question, either in the operating room or postoperatively, is how successful the repair is in abolishing regurgitation. Transesophageal echo has been shown to compare very well with angiography in the assessment of the severity of mitral regurgitation after repair[2]. No, minimal, or 1+ regurgitation is considered a good result. If there is more than 1+ regurgitation, the mechanism of regurgitation should be determined if possible: persistent prolapse or flail, a perforation, restricted motion of a leaflet (segment), systolic anterior motion of the mitral valve, or others. Two factors may lead to overestimation or underestimation of residual mitral regurgitation:
- Very early after cardiopulmonary bypass, there is diffuse left ventricular systolic dysfunction. Some mitral regurgitation may abate after better contraction ensues.
- As always in mitral regurgitation, afterload is crucially important. For a realistic assessment of residual regurgitation, systemic blood pressure has to reach near-normal values. This may be achieved transiently be administrating a vasoconstrictor. It may also be necessary to shut off an intraortic balloon pump, if one was inserted.
With postoperative 1+ or 2+ regurgitation, the decision about further surgery must be individualized, based on the feasibility of achieving a better result, the prolongation of the operation and other factors. The available outcome data from such situations favor a "low threshold for performing further surgery" (3; see below).
With 3+ or 4+ residual regurgitation on the postpump intraoperative echo, the patient is usually a candidate for a second pump run, leading to either repeat repair or valve replacement.
A rare (approximately 5% of repairs, range 2-16%) but dramatic complication of mitral valve repair, which can be uniquely identified by echo, is systolic anterior motion of the mitral leaflets after repair[4-9] (Fig. 1,2). This may conceptually be viewed as the presence of too much leaflet material compared to the decreased ring size, leading to slack in particular of the anterior mitral leaflet and to obstruction of the outflow tract by excess leaflet material. The obstruction may be severe, with septal contact of the anterior leaflet in systole, maximal gradients up to 100 mmHg or more, and systemic hypotension. Simultaneously, this complication leads to severe mitral regurgitation. As in hypertrophic obstructive cardiomyopathy, the administration of catecholamines to increase inotropy and cardiac output leads to a deleterious vicious circle. Instead, massive volume expansion and cautious use of a beta-adrenergic blocker are beneficial. If sufficiently severe the situation requires repeat surgery, using "sliding leaflet" techniques or even valve replacement[6,7]. Table 2 enumerates factors predisposing to the postoperative development of SAM. The most important of these factors seems to be the height of the posterior leaflet, especially if associated with a relatively low height of the anterior leaflet and a low distance of the mitral coaptation point to the septum. A recent study[9] comparing patients with post-repair SAM to patients without development of SAM found a preoperative leaflet length (insertion to coaptation point) of 2.2±0.4 cm vs. 1.4±0.3 cm, a ratio of anterior to posterior to anterior leaflet length of 1±0.1 vs. 2±0.5 and a distance of the coaptation point to the septum of 2.5±0.3 vs. 3.0±0.6 cm, respectively.

Mitral stenosis created by valve repair is very uncommon. However, some such instances have been recognized. Especially in young children undergoing repair for congenital mitral regurgitation (e.g., endocardial cushion defects) or in patients with preexisting rheumatic disease this complication occurs.

POSTOPERATIVE EVALUATION OF MITRAL VALVE REPLACEMENT

Both bioprosthetic and mechanical prostheses are very well evaluated by echo; while the atrial side is obscured in mechanical prostheses viewed by transthoracic echo by the typical reverberation artifacts, transesophageal echo offers a superb, close look at the atrial side. This is important since thrombotic or endocarditic mass lesions (vegetations) tend to adhere to the atrial side of prostheses. Usually, the movement of the occluder or the leaflets can be seen in sufficient detail to determine whether there is structural integrity or abnormal obstruction. Furthermore, abnormal rocking of the prosthesis during the heart cycle due to partial dehiscence may be detected.

Doppler mean gradients may be obtained both by transthoracic and transesophageal echo. As a rule of thumb, mean gradients at normal heart rates and in the absence of a hyperdynamic circulation do not exceed 5 ± 3 mmHg in mitral valve prostheses. Of course, the caveats for using gradients to assess obstruction apply; for example, in severely depressed left ventricular function with low stroke volume, an obstruction may be masked by a normal gradient. Direct evidence of normal occluder motion should therefore always be sought. In the presence of bileaflet valves, it should be remembered that there are somewhat higher velocities and hence gradients across the central orifice than across the side orifices, due to valve design. The side orifice velocities are approximately 85% of the central orifice velocity, and approximately one third of the maximal pressure drop across the central orifice (corresponding to the central orifice velocity) is recovered in the mitral position[10]. On average, even the peak calculated gradients across the central orifice are only about 2 mmHg higher than the gradients across the side orifices.

The use of the pressure half-time method to assess the mitral valve orifice area in the presence of a prosthesis is meaningful only if serial measurements are compared. Prosthetic design affects the pressure half-time significantly, and thus the formula A=220/PHT (A orifice area in cm², PHT pressure half-time in ms) cannot be applied. However, obstruction will prolong pressure half-time in comparison to baseline values. Furthermore, an increase in transprosthetic flow due to severe regurgitation affects pressure half-time less than it affects transprosthetic gradients. Thus, serial measurements of pressure half-time may allow to sort out whether an increased gradient is due to the presence of new regurgitation or if there is additional obstruction.

The evaluation of prosthetic regurgitation by transthoracic echo is difficult due to the reduced acoustic accessibility of the left atrium. Helpful maneuvers are
- the careful use of parasternal and subcostal views to evaluate the left atrium by color Doppler
- attention to the presence of proximal convergence zones on the left ventricular side of the prosthesis, indicating indirectly the presence of substantial regurgitation.

Again, transesophageal echocardiography offers excellent access to the "back side" of the prosthesis. In particular, it allows better differentiation of transprosthetic normal and abnormal regurgitation[11,12] and of paravalvular leaks. Placing the prosthesis in the center of the color Doppler sector, and rotating the cross-section in small increments across the whole arc to 180° allows complete scanning of the valvular circumference, ensuring that no eccentric jet is missed. Also, assessment of pulmonary venous flow[13,14] and use of the proximal convergence zone for evaluation of severity can be performed from the transesophageal window[15].

In the immediate postoperative setting (coming off cardiopulmonary bypass), the severity of paravalvular leaks, which are relatively common and sometimes multiple, should be assessed with caution. As indicated above for mitral valve repair, realistic load conditions (in particular near-normal systolic blood pressure) have to be established to assess regurgitation. Also, a recent study found that some paravalvular leaks disappear and others decrease their color Doppler jet area after reversal of anticoagulation by protamine[16], especially in mechanical mitral valve prostheses (Fig.3). Final judgement might therefore be postponed until after reversal of anticoagulation, except for torrential paravalvular leakage or clear valve dehiscence.

OTHER TYPICAL POSTOPERATIVE PROBLEMS

A. *Left ventricular function*
Left ventricular function in mitral stenosis typically is good and remains good after surgery. In contrast, left ventricular function in mitral regurgitation is often impaired and may further deteriorate immediately postoperatively. Reasons for this deterioration include:

1) Coming off cardiopulmonary bypass there is a short period of global hypokinesia, which usually resolves within minutes.
2) Acutely increased afterload by removing regurgitation. This is especially true for not dilated left ventricles, leading to a decrease in ejection fraction postoperatively. Although in chronic severe mitral regurgitation with left ventricular dilatation ultimately afterload decreases, because the left ventricle decreases in size and so does systolic wall stress, in the acute postoperative phase there may also be some deterioration of global left ventricular function.
3) Underfilling of the left ventricle (volume depletion). Typically, the left ventricle shows cavity obliteration in end-systole and the right ventricle is small.
4) Loss of longitudinal shortening by severing the subvalvular chordal apparatus in valve replacement. Newer techniques attempt to avoid this preserving valvulo-ventricular continuity at least in part by reinsertion of chordae.

5) Ischemia by postoperative air-embolism to the coronaries (typically to the right coronary artery) or direct damage of a coronary artery. In particular, the circumflex artery, which courses in the atrioventricular groove may be damaged during surgery. In the presence of coronary artery disease, acute occlusion of a vessel can also occur spontaneously. The hallmark of coronary ischemia is a regional wall motion abnormality. Ischemia by air-embolism usually resolves completely within minutes.

6) Finally, hypoxemia, acidosis, electrolyte shifts or arrhythmia have to be considered.

B. *Aortic dissection*

This rare complication originates from the cannulation site, typically the ascending aorta. The postoperative transesophageal echo should therefore include (as all transesophageal echos should) a look at the ascending and descending aorta.

C. *Right sided problems*

There is controversy over what amount of concomitant tricuspid regurgitation constitutes an indication for surgical intervention, usually an annuloplasty with a ring. Although it is notoriously difficult to assess tricuspid regurgitation intraoperatively by transesophageal echo, an effort should be made to estimate the severity after mitral valve surgery, when previously high pulmonary pressures are presumably lowered. This is also an important point in the pre-discharge echo.

DOES THE POSTOPERATIVE ECHO MAKE A DIFFERENCE?

It is clear that severe complications such as persistent severe mitral regurgitation after repair or large paravalvular leaks after valve replacement can be readily detected by intraoperative echo and treated while the chest is still open. It is less clear where the threshold for a second pump run lies in the presence of mild-to-moderate post-repair regurgitation.

Data from the Cleveland Clinic[2] indicate that in the presence of 1+ to 2+ regurgitation post-repair there is a trend towards more frequent late reoperations in such patients. Comparing 76 patients with 1+ or 2+ post-repair regurgitation to matched patients with no post-repair regurgitation, this study found a higher rate of re-operations over the next four years in the "less than echo-perfect" group (Fig.4).

In a recent large retrospective analysis of 1072 patients undergoing mitral valve repair for degenerative disease at the same institution[17], the use of intraoperative echo was found to be a significant predictor for freedom from reoperation in subsequent years in a multivariate model of risk factors for reoperation (Fig.5).

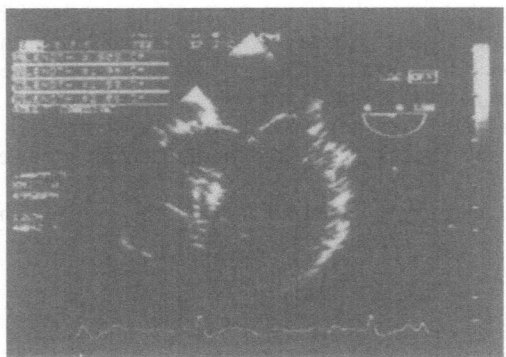

Figure 1: Images of a patient developing postoperative systolic anterior motion (SAM) of the mitral valve after repair. Top: preoperative image. No SAM is present. Middle: pronounced SAM with septal contact. Bottom: resolution of SAM after discontinuation of catecholamines, administration of volume, vasopressors and a beta-blocker (esmolol). Reproduced with permission from Maslow AD et al., Echocardiographic predictors of left ventricular outflow tract obstruction and systolic anterior motion of the mitral valve after mitral valve reconstruction for myxomatous valve disease. J Am Coll Cardiol 1999;34: 2096-104

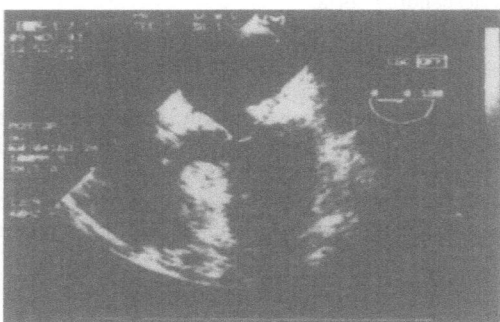

Figure 2: Schematic drawing indicating linear measurements important in the prediction of postoperative SAM. C coaptation point, AML anterior leaflet length, PML posterior leaflet length, SEP-C distance from coaptation point to septum. See text for further details.

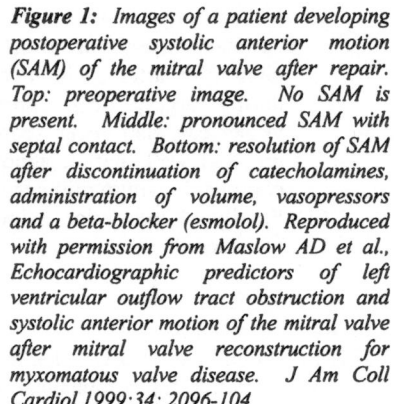

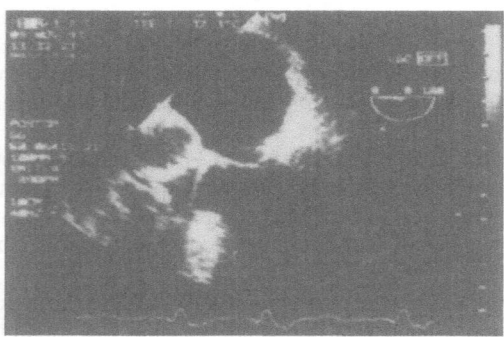

Figure 3: Intraoperative, post-pump images of a mitral bioprosthesis in the transverse (0°) plane before (left) and after (right) protamine reversal of anticoagulation. The number of regurgitant jets decreases from three to one. Reproduced with permission from Morehead et al., Intraoperative echocardiographic detection of regurgitant jets after valve replacement, Ann Thorac Surg 2000;69:135-9.

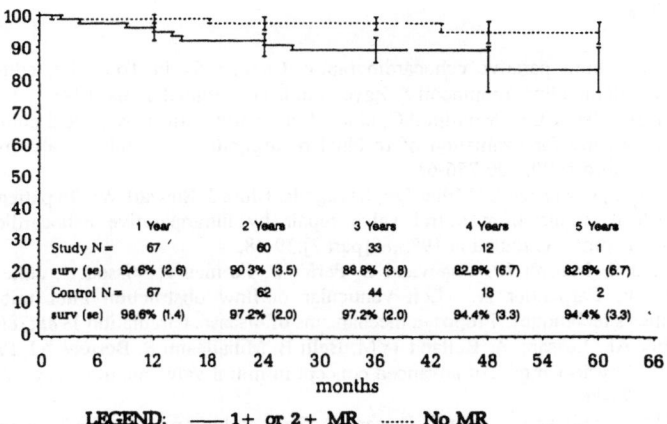

LEGEND: —— 1+ or 2+ MR ······· No MR

Figure 4: *Kaplan-Meier curve showing freedom from reoperation for recurrent mitral regurgitation (MR) after mitral repair in the study group with 1+ or 2+ MR compared with the control group with no MR by postpump echocardiography. Reproduced with permission from Fix J et al., Do patients with less than 'echo-perfect' results from mitral valve repair by intraoperative echocardiography have a different outcome? Circulation 1993,88[part 2]:39-48.*

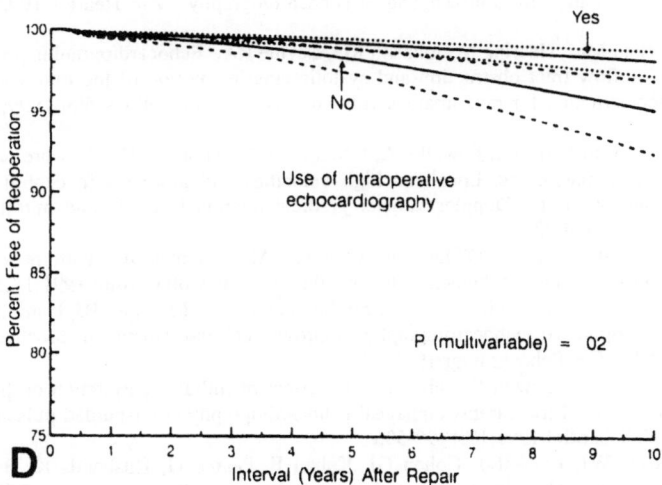

Figure 5: *Influence of intraoperative echocardiography versus no intraoperative echocardiography on freedom from reoperation. The presentation is a risk-adjusted comparison using a multivariate model. Reproduced with permission from Gillinov AM et al, Durability of mitral valve repair for degenerative disease. J Thorac Cardiovasc surg 1998; 116:734-43*

66

REFERENCES

1. Stewart WJ. Intraoperative echocardiography. Chapter 54 in Topol EJ, editor: Textbook of Cardiovascular medine, Lippincott & Raven Publishers, Philadelphia, 1998
2. Reichert SL, Visser CA, Moulijn AC, et al. Intraopertive transeoshpageal color-coded Doppler ehcocardiography for evaluation of residual regurgitation after mitral valve repair. J Thorac Cardiovasc Surg 1990; 100:756-61
3. Fix J, Isada L, Cosgrove D, Miller DP, Savage R, Blum J, Stewart W: Do patients with less than 'echo-perfect' results from mitral valve repair by intraoperative echocardiography have a different outcome ? Circulation 1993,88[part 2]:39-48.
4. Mihaileanu S, Marino JP, Chauvaud S, Perier P, Forman J, Vissoat J, Julien J, Dreyfus G, Abastado P, Carpentier A. Left venticular outflow obstruction after mitral valve repair (Carpentier's technique). Proposed mechanisms of disease. Circulation 1988;78(Suppl.1):78-84.
5. Carpentier AF, Lessana A, Relland JYM, Belli E, Mihaileanu S, Berrebi AJ, Palsky E, Loumet DF. The "Physio-Ring": An advanced concept in mitral valve annuloplasty. Ann Thorac Surg 1995;60:1177-86
6. Jebara VA, Mihaileanu S, Acar C, Brizard C, Grare P, Latremouille C, Chauvaud S, Fabiani JN, Deloche A, Carpentier A. Left ventricular outflow tract obstruction after mitral valve repair. Results of the sliding leaflet technique. Circulation 1993;88(part2): 30-34
7. Lee KS, Stewart WJ, Lever HM, Underwood PL, Cosgrove DM: Mechanism of outflow tract obstruction causing failed mitral valve repair. Anterior displacement of leaflet coaptation. Circulation 1993,88[part 2]:24-29
8. Webster PJ, Raper RF, Ross DE, Edwards AC, Choong CY: Pharmacologic abolition of severe mitral regurgitation associated with dynamic left ventricular outflow tract obstruction after mitral valve repair: Confirmation by transesophageal echocardiography. Am Heart J 1993,126:480-483.
9. Maslow AD, Regan MM, Haering M, Johnson RG, Levine RA. Echocardiographic predictors of left ventricular outflow tract obstruction and systolic anterior motion of the mitral valve after mitral valve reconstruction for myxomatous valve disease. J Am Coll Cardiol 1999;34: 2096-104
10. Vandervoort PM, Greenberg NL, Powell KA, Cosgrove DM, Thomas JD. Pressure recovery in bileaflet heart valve prostheses. Localized high velocities and gradients in central and side orifices with implications for Doppler-catheter gradient relation in aortic and mitral position. Circulation 1995;92:3474-72.
11. Flachskampf FA, Guerrero JL, O'Shea JP, Weyman AE, Thomas JD. Patterns of normal transvalvular regurgitation in mechanical valve prostheses. J Am Coll Cardiol 1991;18:1493-8
12. Flachskampf FA, Hoffmann R, Franke A, Job FP, Schöndube FA, Messmer BJ, Hanrath P. Does multiplane transesophageal echocardiography improve the assessment of prosthetic valve regurgitation ? J Am Soc Echocardiogr 1995;8:70-8
13. Castello R, Pearson AC, Lenzen P, Labovitz AJ. Effect of mitral regurgitation on pulmonary venous velocities derived from transesophageal echocardiography color-guided pulsed Doppler imaging. J Am Coll Cardiol 1991;17:1499-506
14. Klein AL, Stewart WJ, Bartlett J, Cohen GI, Kahan F, Pearce G, Husbands K, Bailey AS, Salcedo EE, Cosgrove DM. Effects of mitral regurgitation on pulmonary venous flow and left atrial pressure: An intraoperative transesophageal echocardiographic study. J Am Coll Cardiol 1992;20:1345-52.
15. Flachskampf FA, Frieske R, Engelhard B, Grenner H, Frielingsdorf J, Beck F, Reineke T, Thomas JD, Hanrath P. Comparison of transesophageal Doppler methods with angiography for evaluation of the severity of mitral regurgitation. J Am Soc Echocardiogr 1998;11:882-92

16. Morehead AJ, Firstenberg MS, Shiota T, Quin J, Armstrong G, Cosgrove DM III, Thomas JD. Intraoperative echocardiographic detection of regurgitant jets after valve replacement. Ann Thorac Surg 2000; 69:135-9

17. Gillinov AM, Cosgrove DM, Blackstone EH, Diaz R, Arnold JH, Lytle BW, Smedira NG, Sabik JF, McCarthy PM, Loop FD. Durability of mitral valve repair for degenerative disease. J Thorac Cardiovasc Surg 1998; 116:734-43

Checklist for the postoperative evaluation after mitral valve surgery

- Is there native or prosthetic mitral regurgitation, how severe is it, and what is the mechanism ?
- In native valves: residual prolapse or flail, restricted leaflet motion, lack of coaptation due to dilatation, perforation/destruction.
- In prostheses: normal transvalvular / paraprosthetic / abnormal transvalvular regurgitation, rocking of the valve as a sign of dehiscence.
- Is there mitral stenosis or prosthetic obstruction ?
- How is global left ventricular systolic function ?
- Are there new regional wall motion abnormalities (in particular posteriorly or inferiorly) ?
- Is there systolic anterior motion (SAM) of the mitral valve (after repair)?
- Are there generic complications of cardiac surgery (pericardial effusion, aortic dissection) ?

Factors predisposing for the development of systolic anterior motion of the mitral valve after repair of mitral regurgitation[5-7,9]

- Increased height and excess tissue of posterior leaflet
- Small valvuloplasty ring
- Reduced distance from mitral leaflet coaptation point to septum (more anterior coaptation point)
- Relatively small ventricle, relatively large mitral leaflets
- Rigid prosthetic ring ? (debated in the literature)
- Narrow angle inflow / outflow tract ? (debated in the literature)

Section III / Chapter 1

PREOPERATIVE EVALUATION OF AORTIC INSUFFICIENCY: OPTIMAL TIMING

C.H. PEELS

INTRODUCTION

As in mitral regurgitation, optimal timing of surgical intervention in aortic regurgitation remains challenging and controversial. Both conditions deal with volume overload, but in aortic regurgitation there is evident combined overload of volume and pressure imposed on the left ventricle[1-3].

In aortic regurgitation forward cardiac output is maintained by an increase of the total stroke volume, an increase corresponding to the severity of regurgitation. This increase in total stroke volume is achieved by ventricular dilation. This increased stroke volume has to be ejected into the high impedance aorta leading to a left ventricular pressure overload as well. The left ventricle keeps end-systolic wall stress, a measure for left ventricular afterload, in the normal range by matching dilation with an increase in wall thickness. During progression of the disease, the degree of wall thickening fails to keep pace with left ventricular dilation and wall stress rises. At this time-point hemodynamic decompensation follows with as the first sign a fall in ejection performance related to this increased afterload. Therefore, after surgical correction meaning removal of this excess in afterload, ejection performance should normalize. However, continued overload can lead to depression of contractility and these patients are less likely to improve after surgical intervention.

In the asymptomatic patient, the challenge lies in appropriate timing of surgery in which the benefit of preserving contractile dysfunction has to be weighted against the risks of surgery and the possession of a valve prosthesis. Besides assessment of the cause and severity of the regurgitant lesion, for pre-operative evaluation, measurements of left ventricular function are pivotal since patients with chronic severe aortic regurgitation typically remain asymptomatic for extended periods of time and progression to contractile dysfunction may precede symptom onset[4].

ETIOLOGY OF AORTIC REGURGITATION

Echocardiography can provide reliable information on anatomy of the aortic valve and root and allows identification of the mechanism of regurgitation.

Primary pathologic abnormalities of the aortic valve leaflets account for 2/3 of patients with chronic aortic regurgitation and dilation of the aortic root and a combination of valve and root abnormality for the other 1/3 of patients. Acute severe aortic regurgitation is most often caused by endocarditis, aortic dissection or trauma.

For follow-up of patients with severe regurgitation, the etiology is of importance. For example, in aortic root disease surgical timing not only depends on the development of left ventricular changes due to chronic overload but also and in some patients moreover depends on rate and extent of root dilation. In Marfan's syndrome the degree of aortic root dilation is an important clinical risk factor for dissection[5,6]. The rate of progression of root dilation is variable and the root dimension should be related to age and body surface area[7]. The aortic root ratio (= actual sinus dimension/predicted sinus dimension) can be used to identify in Marfan patients a lower risk group: when this ratio is less than 1.3 and the annual change in the ratio less than 5%, no complications occurred in this series of 89 consecutive patients[5].

Diseases as this, aortic root dilation, and bicuspid aortic valve tend to progress and lead to increase in regurgitant severity. These patients should be followed more closely for development of severe aortic regurgitation with sequellae for the left ventricle than patients with mild to moderate regurgitation caused by other etiology.

ASSESSMENT OF SEVERITY OF AORTIC REGURGITATION

Doppler and two-dimensional echocardiographic examination give, besides the anatomic information on the valve, also the parameters to quantify the severity of regurgitation. Furthermore, echocardiography provides precise and reproducible measures of left ventricular dimensions and function, the keystone in decision making for follow up and eventually for surgery.

Color flow evaluation of regurgitant severity has become a standard clinical technique and is valid for differentiating minimal from moderate or severe regurgitation. Perhaps the most useful view for this purpose is the parasternal short axis view just on the ventricular side of the aortic leaflets: every trivial jet is noticed, multiple jets can be seen and the regurgitant area in relation to the outflowtract area can be estimated or measured. Semiquantitative grading of severity can be done with color flow Doppler, corresponding to the semiquantitative angiographic grading, as: **grade 1+** : trivial or mild: color flow jet limited to the region immediately adjacent to valve closure, may not be seen at every beat (trivial), **grade 2+** : mild to moderate: color flow jet filling up to one third of the left ventricle and seen on every beat, **grade 3+** : moderate to severe: color flow reaching and filling up to two third of the left ventricle and seen on every beat, and **grade 4+** : severe: color flow reaching the apex of the left ventricle and almost filling most of the ventricle, flow reversal present in the descending aorta. Grade 1+ and 2+ are usually considered as being less than surgical severity and grade 3+ and 4+ to be of surgical severity.

Therefore, for practical reasons in non-invasive imaging grading is done in mild (including trivial), moderate and severe, where severe is grade 3+ and 4+ (8).

Assessment of this grade has to be done in at least two orthogonal image planes and the extent of the flow disturbance in these views has to be integrated.

A useful parameter when using color flow imaging to grade aortic regurgitation is the ratio of the color flow jet height at aortic valve level (the vena contracta) to the width of the left ventricular outflow tract. This visualization of the vena contracta quantifies in a very real sence the regurgitant orifice area. When this ratio stays under 0,25, this corresponds to a mild aortic regurgitation, when the ratio reaches 45-50% this is consistent with moderate regurgitation and a ratio above 50-60% always indicates a severe regurgitation[9].

Holodiastolic flow reversal in the aortic arch or descending aorta is one of the most useful signs of significant aortic regurgitation. The most sensitive sign in this respect is holodiastolic flow reversal in the proximal abdominal aorta, always indicating severe aortic regurgitation[10].

In systole, aortic regurgitation is associated with a small transvalvular pressure gradient unless coexisting aortic stenosis is present, which is not infrequent. In diastole, the aortic diastolic pressure decreases more rapidly than normal which can be detected in a relatively low diastolic blood pressure. In chonic aortic regurgitation, left ventricular diastolic pressure remains low due to the increased compliance of the dilated left ventricle. Consequently, the time course of the magnitude of the difference between aortic and left ventricular pressures in diastole depends on the severity, the duration and the degree of decompensation of the left ventricle. This diastolic pressure difference is the basis for these non-invasive findings and for the characteristics of the diastolic murmur : in acute regurgitation and decompensated aortic regurgitation due to more rapid equilibration of diastolic pressures a low-pitched, short murmur and in chronic, compensated regurgitation a high-pitched holodiastolic murmur. Equivalent to this murmur, the continuous wave Doppler spectrum of the diastolic transvalvular velocity of flow shows in acute and decompensated aortic regurgitation a steep slope of velocity deceleration and in chronic and compensated regurgitation a more flat slope. A common index to reproduce this slope of diastolic flow velocity is the time required to reach half of the initial aortic-ventricular gradient. This time is given by the time required of the initial aortic regurgitant velocity (the maximal regurgitant velocity) to fall to $1/\sqrt{2}$ or 70.7% of its initial value, this time is called the pressure half-time. Of course this is not a pure measure of regurgitant severity, the value is directly related to aortic and ventricular compliance and the initial gradient. It is a parameter which can be used in the same patient for follow-up.

Exercise testing may be helpful when there is discrepancy between the clinical presentation and the resting echocardiographic findings, when echocardiographic data are non-diagnostic or when indications for surgical intervention in an asymptomatic patient are borderline[11]. The ejection fraction of the left ventricle can be measured at rest and after exercise using 2 dimensional echocardiography or radionuclide techniques, a normal response in compensated aortic regurgitation being an increase in ejection fraction of 5 units or more after exercise[12].

NONINVASIVE FOLLOW UP IN CHRONIC AORTIC REGURGITATION

Central in optimal timing of surgical intervention in patients with chronic aortic regurgitation is periodic non-invasive evaluation since some patients develop irreversible dysfunction of the left ventricle without any clinical symptoms. The timing of follow up must be tailored to each patient depending on the severity of the valve lesion, the cause of regurgitation as mentioned above, and the degree of left ventricular dilation at initial examination. But, since symptoms occur late in the disease, follow up to find the 'golden moment' for surgery has to be protocollized and non-invasive methods are sufficient to do so. Most physicians use 2 dimensional and Doppler echocardiography to evaluate ventricular dimensions and volumes once the lesion severity is assessed.

A mild degree of regurgitation without any abnormality in ventricular dimensions or function does not oblige to frequent examination unless the underlying disease is likely to progress (for example Marfan's syndrome or bicuspid valve lesion).

The patient with moderate to severe aortic regurgitation and mild ventricular dilation should be examined annually with measurement of ventricular dimensions and ejection fraction as long as these parameters remain stable. When an increase in dimension or a fall in ejection fraction is found, a repeat examination on a shorter interval (3-6 months) should be done to differentiate true progressive disease from measurement variability.

Patients with moderate to severe regurgitation and evident left ventricular dilation but still a normal ejection fraction need more intensive follow up. A second examination at 3-6 months can assess if this patient is stable or progresses into the stage where prompt surgical intervention is needed. When there is uncertainty in this matter, exercise testing with measurement of ejection fraction either using 2 dimensional echocardiography or radionuclide techniques may be helpful.

TIMING OF SURGICAL INTERVENTION

Aortic valve surgery should only be considered if the valve lesion is severe. This is an important consideration in patients with combined pathology as coronary artery disease and aortic regurgitation.

Symptomatic patients with normal left ventricular dimensions (endsystolic dimension < 45 mm) and function (ejection fraction > 50%) are considered for surgery if the regurgitation is severe and the clinician is convinced that symtomatology originates from the valve lesion. When there is doubt about the latter, exercise testing may be helpful or a short observational period in which ventricular function is monitored closely. When chamber size increases and systolic function declines even when the threshold values for chamber size and function are not achieved, surgery is indicated.

Symptomatic patients with left ventricular dilation (endsystolic dimension >45-55 mm) and signs of ventricular dysfunction (ejection fraction < 50%) should undergo aortic valve surgery.

Since the majority of symptomatic patients have improved survival, functional class and left ventricular function after aortic valve surgery, regardless of the left ventricular function, all these patients should be referred for surgery. Even in patients with NYHA functional class IV and an ejection fraction of <0.25, the well known high risk of surgical intervention, which approaches the 10%, than the higher risk of medical management[13].

It is generally agreed that valve surgery is indicated in asymptomatic patients when signs of left ventricular dysfunction have developed. This is defined as an ejection fraction below the normal limits, being < 0.50 [14,15]. When severe dilation develops, being endsystolic dimension >55 mm and/or enddiastolic dimension >75 mm, surgery is also recommended in the asymptomatic patient even if the ejection fraction is still within the normal range because they represent a high risk group for sudden death[16], the results of valve surgery are excellent and postoperative mortality is considerable once these patients develop symptoms and/or left ventricular dysfunction [17].

A decrease in the ejection fraction during exercise should not be used in the asymptomatic patient with normal ventricular function at rest to decide for surgery because this response to exercise is multifactorial and the strength of evidence that a high risk group is selected this way is limited[18].

FACTORS INFLUENCING OUTCOME AFTER SURGERY FOR AORTIC REGURGITATION

Survival rates derived from literature from operations done in the 1970's, reflect the results of aortic valve surgery in symptomatic patients and ranged from 55 to 76 % 3 year survival and 48 to 58 % 10 year survival[19,20], rather poor figures. Figures from later years show improvement in survival, 5 year survival rates from 82-83% in the 1980's series [21,22]. Clinical improvement was mostly seen, in 70-80% of operated patients there was improvement in functional class despite NYHA class III or IV or an impaired left ventricular function preoperatively, with around 40% of patients becoming asymptomatic.

Left ventricular function typically improves after aortic valve replacement for aortic regurgitation with correction of the volume overload and elimination of the pressure overload. There is however a subset of patients with persistent left ventricular dysfunction postoperatively indicating irreversible contractile dysfunction and they represent a group of patients with a poor prognosis.

Several clinical predictors as cardio-thoracic ratio > 0.58 on the chest x-ray , age > 65 years[21], marked left ventricular hypertrophy on the electrocardiogram[19], NYHA class III or IV, elevated systolic blood pressure (>140 mmHg) or decreased diastolic pressure (< 40 mmHg) have been described identifying patients at increased risk for postoperative death.

Left ventricular systolic function is in these patients the most important determinant of survival. The indices used to describe left ventricular function are ejection fraction above or below 0.50 and endsystolic left ventricular dimension (LVESD) above or below 55 mm. An ejection fraction of <0.50 portends a significantly poorer 3 year survival, around 64%, than an ejection fraction in the normal range with a survival around 90%, in symptomatic patients[22]. The same holds true for the LVESD: an ESD < 55 mm predicts a much better 3,5 year survival (83%) than > 55 mm (42%)[23]. Other factors influencing outcome are the duration of left ventricular dysfunction, patients with prolonged (>18 months) duration of dysfunction of the left ventricle had a 5 year survival of only 45%, in contrast to those with more brief existing dysfunction, a 100% 5 year survival[24].

Furthermore, the exercise capacity before operation is predictive of outcome: a preserved exercise capacity (duration of exercise > 22,5 min) predicted a very good outcome (100% 3,5 year survival) compared to a survival of 52% in patients with an impaired exercise capacity [4].

IN SUMMARY

In aortic regurgitation, the timing of surgery is relatively straightforward: all symptomatic patients with severe aortic regurgitation benefit from surgery in terms of better functional class, survival and ventricular function postoperatively and should thus be referred for surgery as soon as this valve lesion is diagnosed, regardless of the left ventricular function at that moment. Asymptomatic patients with left ventricular dysfunction develop symptoms in the near future and should be referred for elective aortic relacement. Asymptomatic patients with preserved left ventricular dimensions and function and a normal exercise tolerance should be followed closely with non-invasive measurements of dimensions and ejection fraction. When deterioration of these parameters occur, the robustness of these findings should be confirmed by serial repeated measurements and once dilation and/or dysfunction of the left ventricle are assessed, referral for surgery should take place. The thresholds for unacceptable dilation (LVESD > 45-50 mm) and ejection fraction (< 50-60 %) are somewhat broader than in mitral regurgitation, because improvement postoperatively of left ventricular function and dimensions occurs almost in all patients when duration of these abnormalities was not long which can be obviated when close follow-up is guaranteed.

REFERENCES

1. Carabello BA: Aortic regurgitation. A lesion with similarities to both aortic stenosis and mitral regurgitation. Circulation 1990;82:1051-1053
2. Ross J Jr: Afterload mismatch in aortic and mitral valve disease: implications of surgical therapy. J Am Coll Cardiol 1985;5:811-826
3. Borow KM: Surgical outcome in chronic aortic regurgitation: a physiologic framework for assessing preoperative predictors. J Am Coll Cardiol 1987;10:1165-1170
4. Bonow RO, Rosing DR, Kent KM et al: Timing of operation for chronic aortic regurgitation. Am J Cardiol 1982;50:325-336
5. Legget ME, Unger TA, O'Sullivan CK et al: Aortic root complications in Marfan's syndrome: identification of a lower risk group. Heart 1996;75:389-395
6. Silverman DI, Gray J, Roman MJ et al: Family history of severe cardiovascular disease in Marfan syndrome is associated with increased aortic diameter and decreased survival. J Am Coll Cardiol 1995;26:1062-1067
7. Roman MJ, Deveraux RB, Kramer-Fox R, O'Loughlin J: Two dimensional echocardiographic aortic root dimensions in normal children and adults. Am J Cardiol 1989;64:507-512
8. Otto CM: Echocardiographic evaluation of valvular heart disease in Valvular Heart Disease, Philidelphia: W.B.Saunders 1999:43-79
9. Perry GJ, Helmcke JA, Nanda NC et al: Evaluation of aortic insufficiency by Doppler clor flow mapping. J Am Coll Cardiol 1987;9:962-957
10. Takenaka K, Dabestani A, Gardin JM, Russell D, Clark S, Allfie A, Henry WL: A simple Doppler echocardiographic method for estimating severity of aortic regurgitation. Am J Cardiol 1986;57:1340-1343
11. van den Brink RB, Verheul HA, Hoedemaker G et al: The value of Doppler echocardiography in the management of patients with valvular heart disease: analysis of one year of clinical practice. J Am Soc Echocardiogr 1991;4:109-120
12. Massie BM, Kramer BL, Loge D et al: Ejection fraction response to supine exercise in asymptomatic aortic regurgitation: relation to simultaneous hemodynamic measurements. J Am Coll Cardiol 1985;5:847-855
13. Bonow RO, Nikas D, Elefteriades JA: Valve replacement for regurgitant lesions of the aortic or mitral valve in advanced left ventricular dysfunction. Cardiol Clin 1995;13:73-83
14. Bonow RO,: Aymptomatic aortic regurgitation: indications for operation. J Card Surg 1994;9:170-173
15. Nishimura RA, McGoon MD, Schaff HV, Giuliani ER: Chronic aortic regurgitation: indications for operation-1988. Mayo Clin Proc 1988;63:270-280
16. Turina J, Turina M, Rothlin M, Krayenbuehl HP: Improved late survival in patients with chronic aortic regurgitation by earlier operation. Circulation 1984;70:I:147-152
17. Klodas E, Enriquez-Sarano M, Tajik AJ, Mullany CJ, Bailey KR, Seward JB: Aortic regurgitation complicated by extreme left ventricular dilation: long-term outcome after surgical correction. J Am Coll Cardiol 1996;27:670-677
18. Bonow RO, Picone AL, McIntosh CL, et al: Survival and functional results after valve replacement for aortic regurgitation from 1976 to 1983: impact of preoperative left ventricular function. Circulation 1985;72:1244-1256
19. Roberts DL, DeWeese JA, Mahoney EB et al: Long-term survival following aortic valve replacement. Am Heart J 1976;91:311-317
20. Hirshfeld JW, Epstein SE, Roberts AJ et al: Indices predicting long-term survival after valve replacement in patients with aortic regurgitattion and patients with aortic stenosis. Circulation 1974;50:1190-1199

21. Acar J, Luxereau PH, Ducimentiere P et al: Prognosis of surgically treated chronic aortic valve disease. Predictive indicators of early postoperative risk and long-term survival based on 439 cases. J Thorac cardiovasc Surg 1981;82:114
22. Forman R, Firth BG, Barnard MS: Prognostic significance of preoperative left ventricular ejection fraction and valve lesion in patients with aortic valve replacement. Am J Cardiol 1980;45:1120-1125.
23. Henry WL, Bonow RO, Borer JS et al: Observations on the optimum time for operative intervention for aortic regurgitation. I.Evaluation of the results of aortic valve replacement in symtomatic patients. Circulation 1980;61:471-483
24. Bonow RO, Rosing DR, Maron BJ et al: Reversal of left ventricular dysfunction after aortic valve replacement for chronic aortic regurgitation: Influence of duration of preoperative left ventricular dysfunction. Circulation 1984;70:570-579.

Section III / Chapter 2

HEMODYNAMIC EVALUATION OF AORTIC STENOSIS

Dr. J.M. VAN DANTZIG

INTRODUCTION

With aging of the population, calcific aortic stenosis is becoming a common valvular lesions in clinical practice. Management challenges may present due to advanced age, comorbidity, concomitant coronary artery disease and decreased left ventricular function. For optimal management, information is necessary about valvular morphology and function, left ventricular function and aortic root size.

Cardiac catheterisation traditionally represented the "gold" standard. Using retrograde catheterisation, left ventricular pressure is measured and compared to aortic pressure, preferably recorded simultaneously. The difference between aortic and ventricular pressure may be used as a general indicator of aortic valve stenosis. However, to definitively classify stenosis severity, an estimate of cardiac output should be obtained and aortic valve area calculated[1]. To this end, either the thermodilution method using pulmonary artery catheterisation may be used or Fick's method with direct measurement of arterial and central venous oxygen content and total body oxygen consumption.

However, catheterisation for assessing aortic stenosis has drawbacks. Firstly, it is invasive and associated with mortality and morbidity. In a series of 457 patients with invasive evaluation of aortic stenosis over 11 years, a 1.1% mortality was observed[2]. Secondly, with increasing emphasis on coronary disease in catheterisation laboratories, experience in valvular disease is decreasing. This limits the confidence with which hemodynamics may be used. Of course, disappearance of patients with valve disease from the catheterisation laboratory results from the ascent of echocardiography,[3] which is nowadays the examination of choice in evaluating aortic stenosis and has supplanted invasive hemodynamic evaluation in most centres.

Although a powerful method, a drawback of echocardiography is operator-dependence both in performing the examination and in its interpretation. Since important (surgical) decisions are made based on the echocardiogram solely, it should be performed and interpreted judiciously by personnel with proper skill and experience. Furthermore, in surgical cases, the echocardiogram should be reviewed by the consulting cardiac surgeon, who hence needs to be qualified in interpretation.

ECHOCARDIOGRAPHIC EVALUATION OF AORTIC STENOSIS: ASSESSMENT OF VALVE MORPHOLOGY

Echocardiographic evaluation of aortic stenosis starts by inspecting valve morphology by two-dimensional scanning in multiple views. Valve leaflet number and motion and presence and pattern of calcification should be noted in order to delineate causative pathology and obtain a first impression of stenosis severity. Some have advocated using the two-dimensional (transesophageal) echocardiogram to directly estimate aortic valve area by planimetry in the valve short axis [4;5]. Others however have met with more limited success using this approach[6]. Careful interpretation of the two-dimensional echocardiogram may also reveal non-valvular obstruction (e.g. dynamic or fixed subvalvular left ventricular outflow obstruction, supravalvular obstruction). Furthermore, the two-dimensional echocardiogram may delineate aortic dilatation, necessitating additional surgery. To image the proximal ascending aorta, use of the parasternal long axis view with the transducer shifted one intercostal space cranially from the position used to image the heart is often useful. Finally, measurement of the left ventricular outflow tract diameter is important for aortic valve area calculation, and also may identify patients in whom only a small diameter prosthetic valve can be implanted with the potential for patient-valve mismatch [7]. This may be an important element in selecting the type of prosthesis.

Additionally, left ventricular size and function and the presence and type of left ventricular hypertrophy should be noted. This is important in estimating surgical risk, and may also predict occurrence of dynamic left ventricular outflow obstruction post-operatively [8].

ECHOCARDIOGRAPHIC EVALUATION OF AORTIC STENOSIS: ASSESSMENT OF STENOSIS SEVERITY

This careful two-dimensional examination is then extended by Doppler echocardiography, an accurate estimator of stenosis severity [9-11]. Using continuous wave Doppler, blood velocity across the valve is measured and the pressure gradient calculated with the modified Bernoulli equation ($\Delta P = 4\Delta V^2$). Accuracy is greatly influenced by the care with which the velocity signals are obtained. Highest velocities should be carefully searched, using not only the apical window but also exploring right parasternal and suprasternal approaches. The audio signal supplied by the ultrasound scanner is indispensable in ensuring high quality Doppler spectral displays. By tracing the envelope of this spectrum, maximal and mean pressure gradients may be estimated. Of these, the mean gradients show the least variability [12;13]. A mean gradient of > 50 mmHg is assumed to indicate severe stenosis. In some centres, Doppler signals in patients with poor echo quality is enhanced by administration of a contrast agent [14].

In some patients, Doppler aortic gradients may be considerably higher than catheter gradients. This is explained by pressure recovery [15] [16-20]. Usually, potential energy (pressure) upstream from the valve is dissipated across the stenotic valve and converted completely to heat. However, depending on downstream (aortic root) geometry, aortic valve area and jet direction, flow streamlines may reform and kinetic energy recovered again, resulting in rising pressure distal to the valve. Thus, Doppler estimates of pressure gradients (based on maximal flow velocities) may overestimate catheter gradients (measured distal from the zone of pressure recovery). In one clinical study, a maximal difference of 75 mmHg was demonstrated between Doppler and catheter maximal gradient. Pressure recovery is mainly a problem small aortic roots since the small diameter facilitates reformation of streamlines. In an *in vitro* study, pressure recovery did not occur in aortic roots larger than 30 mm [19]. Also, pressure recovery occurred more readily in moderate as compared to severe stenosis.

Similar to the invasive approach, consideration of stroke volume is important to quantify stenosis severity, especially in patients with decreased left ventricular function or aortic regurgitation [21]. Using the continuity equation, aortic valve area is calculated [10;22;23]. Left ventricular stroke volume is calculated based on the outflow tract diameter in the parasternal long axis view and the flow velocity integral with pulsed Doppler in the apical long axis view. When this is divided by the velocity integral of maximal aortic flow by continuous wave Doppler, aortic valve area is obtained. Values of < 1.0 cm^2 generally indicate severe stenosis. The biggest practical problem with this method is accurate measurement of outflow tract diameter in patients with poor image quality [24-26]. Therefore, the ratio of outflow tract to maximal aortic flow velocity may be used as a rough approximation of severity, [26] with an approximate value of < 0.25 signifying severe stenosis. Another simplification of the continuity equation is substitution of maximal flow velocities for flow integrals. [27]

ASSESSMENT OF STENOSIS SEVERITY IN LOW-FLOW STATES

In most cases, assessment of aortic stenosis is straightforward. However, in "low-flow" states with decreased left ventricular function, several mistakes may be made. Gradients alone must not be relied upon to interpret stenosis severity, since these may be misleadingly low in the setting of severe stenosis, due to low stroke volume. To resolve this issue, calculation of aortic valve area appears an attractive solution. However, aortic valve area both by Gorlin and continuity equation are positively related to absolute flow rate across the valve, implying underestimation of valve area in low flow states [28] [29-35]. One explanation for this underestimation has been offered in a numerical model [32]. A more parabolic flow profile in the vena contracta was shown in low flow states due to increased viscous interaction between the jet and the surrounding walls. Thus, overestimation of the mean maximal flow velocity in the vena contracta occurred, resulting in underestimation of valve area by continuity equation. Another explanation is true increase of anatomic valve area with increasing flow, the valve being more "pushed open" at higher flow rates.

Recently, intriguing data was published which suggested a relation between valve anatomy and the propensity for flow dependence of valve area [36].
Several methods have been suggested to accurately assess low-flow aortic stenosis. Firstly, aortic valve resistance has been suggested to be less dependent on flow rate and may thus represent a more reliable marker of stenosis severity in this situation.[28;31;37-43]. It is calculated by dividing mean systolic pressure gradient by mean systolic flow (= stroke

volume divided by ejection period) with a conversion factor of 1333 to obtain metric unit of dynes*sec*cm^{-5} [41].

Another solution is manipulation of flow rate by dobutamine. The appropriateness of the hemodynamic response should be documented by calculation of stroke volume and cardiac output as dobutamine is increased in 5 ug/kg/min increments every 3–5 minutes and the severity of aortic stenosis judged using the values at the highest dobutamine dose (generally 20 ug/kg/min) [31;44-48].

Even using such techniques, proper patient selection may be difficult but is extremely important, since only patients with severe aortic stenosis in whom left ventricular function is depressed due to afterload mismatch may be expected to recover left ventricular function postoperatively [48-50] and all others would thus be subjected to the high surgical risk of valve replacement in poor ventricular function without the prospect of subsequent recovery of contractile function. Integration of all clinical and echocardiographic data is necessary to arrive at the correct management advice in individual cases [34].

CONCLUSION

Thus, in almost all patients evaluated for surgical replacement of a stenotic aortic valve the echocardiogram provides sufficient pre-operative data. The only role for the catheterisation laboratory in these patients is in defining coronary anatomy and the necessity of concomitant coronary arterial surgery. In cases where complete echocardiographic data is available, retrograde catheterisation of the left ventricle can not be justified.

REFERENCES

1. Gorlin, R and Gorlin, SG. Hydraulic formula for calculation of the area of the stenotic mitral valve, other cardiac valves, and central circulatory shunts. Am.Heart J. 41, 1-29. 1951. Ref Type: Generic

2. Bartsch B, Haase KK, Voelker W, Schobel WA, Karsch KR. [Risk of invasive diagnosis with retrograde catheterization of the left ventricle in patients with acquired aortic valve stenosis][Risiko der invasiven Diagnostik mit retrograder Sondierung des linken Ventrikels bei Patienten mit erworbener Aortenklappenstenose.]. Z.Kardiol. 1999;1999 Apr;88:255-60.

3. Roger VL, Tajik AJ, Reeder GS, Hayes SN, Mullany CJ, Bailey KR et al. Effect of Doppler echocardiography on utilization of hemodynamic cardiac catheterization in the preoperative evaluation of aortic stenosis [see comments]. Mayo Clin.Proc. 1996;1996 Feb;71:141-49.

4. Okura H, Yoshida K, Hozumi T, Akasaka T, Yoshikawa J. Planimetry and transthoracic two-dimensional echocardiography in noninvasive assessment of aortic valve area in patients with valvular aortic stenosis. J.Am.Coll.Cardiol. 1997;1997 Sep;30:753-59.

5. Tribouilloy C, Shen WF, Peltier M, Mirode A, Rey JL, Lesbre JP. Quantitation of aortic valve area in aortic stenosis with multiplane transesophageal echocardiography: comparison with monoplane transesophageal approach. Am.Heart J. 1994;1994 Sep;128:526-32.

6. Bernard Y, Meneveau N, Vuillemenot A, Magnin D, Anguenot T, Schiele F et al. Planimetry of aortic valve area using multiplane transoesophageal echocardiography is not a reliable method for assessing severity of aortic stenosis. Heart 1997;1997 Jul;78:68-73.

7. Rahimtoola SH. Valve prosthesis-patient mismatch: an update [editorial; comment]. J.Heart Valve Dis. 1998;1998 Mar;7:207-10.

8. Bartunek J, Sys SU, Rodrigues AC, van Schuerbeeck E, Mortier L, De Bruyne B. Abnormal systolic intraventricular flow velocities after valve replacement for aortic stenosis. Mechanisms, predictive factors, and prognostic significance. Circulation 1996;1996 Feb 15;93:712-19.

9. Hatle L. Noninvasive assessment and differentiation of left ventricular outflow obstruction with Doppler ultrasound. Circulation 1981;1981 Aug;64:381-87.

10. Skjaerpe T, Hegrenaes L, Hatle L. Noninvasive estimation of valve area in patients with aortic stenosis by Doppler ultrasound and two-dimensional echocardiography. Circulation 1985;1985 Oct;72:810-18.

11. Currie PJ, Seward JB, Reeder GS, Vlietstra RE, Bresnahan DR, Bresnahan JF et al. Continuous-wave Doppler echocardiographic assessment of severity of calcific aortic stenosis: a simultaneous Doppler-catheter correlative study in 100 adult patients. Circulation 1985;1985 Jun;71:1162-69.

12. Panidis IP, Mintz GS, Ross J. Value and limitations of Doppler ultrasound in the evaluation of aortic stenosis: a statistical analysis of 70 consecutive patients. Am.Heart J. 1986;1986 Jul;112:150-58.

13. Krafchek J, Robertson JH, Radford M, Adams D, Kisslo J. A reconsideration of Doppler assessed gradients in suspected aortic stenosis. Am.Heart J. 1985;1985 Oct;110:765-73.

14. Becher H, von Bibra H. [Enhancement of Doppler signals in aortic and mitral valve diseases] [Verstarkung von Doppler-Signalen bei Aorten- und Mitralvitien.]. Z.Kardiol. 1997;1997 Dec;86:1033-39.

15. Levine RA, Jimoh A, Cape EG, McMillan S, Yoganathan AP, Weyman AE. Pressure recovery distal to a stenosis: potential cause of gradient "overestimation" by Doppler echocardiography. J.Am.Coll.Cardiol. 1989;13:706-15.

16. Baumgartner H, Stefenelli T, Niederberger J, Schima H, Maurer G. "Overestimation" of catheter gradients by Doppler ultrasound in patients with aortic stenosis: a predictable manifestation of pressure recovery. J.Am.Coll.Cardiol. 1999;1999 May;33:1655-61.

17. Chambers J. Is pressure recovery an important cause of "Doppler aortic stenosis" with no gradient at cardiac catheterisation? [editorial]. Heart 1996;1996 Nov;76:381-83.
18. Laskey WK, Kussmaul WG. Pressure recovery in aortic valve stenosis. Circulation 1994;1994 Jan;89:116-21.
19. Niederberger J, Schima H, Maurer G, Baumgartner H. Importance of pressure recovery for the assessment of aortic stenosis by Doppler ultrasound. Role of aortic size, aortic valve area, and direction of the stenotic jet in vitro. Circulation 1996;1996 Oct 15;94:1934-40.
20. Schobel WA, Voelker W, Haase KK, Karsch KR. Extent, determinants and clinical importance of pressure recovery in patients with aortic valve stenosis [see comments]. Eur.Heart J. 1999;1999 Sep;20:1355-63.
21. Grayburn PA, Smith MD, Harrison MR, Gurley JC, De Maria AN. Pivotal role of aortic valve area calculation by the continuity equation for Doppler assessment of aortic stenosis in patients with combined aortic stenosis and regurgitation. Am.J.Cardiol. 1988;1988 Feb 1;61:376-81.
22. Oh JK, Taliercio CP, Holmes DR, Jr., Reeder GS, Bailey KR, Seward JB et al. Prediction of the severity of aortic stenosis by Doppler aortic valve area determination: prospective Doppler-catheterization correlation in 100 patients. J.Am.Coll.Cardiol. 1988;1988 Jun;11:1227-34.
23. Zoghbi WA, Farmer KL, Soto JG, Nelson JG, Quinones MA. Accurate noninvasive quantification of stenotic aortic valve area by Doppler echocardiography. Circulation 1986;1986 Mar;73:452-59.
24. Bartunek J, De Bacquer D, Rodrigues AC, De Bruyne B. Accuracy of aortic stenosis severity assessment by Doppler echocardiography: importance of image quality. Int.J.Card Imaging 1995;1995 Jun;11:97-104.
25. Myreng Y, Molstad P, Endresen K, Ihlen H. Reproducibility of echocardiographic estimates of the area of stenosed aortic valves using the continuity equation. Int.J.Cardiol. 1990;1990 Mar;26:349-54.
26. Geibel A, Gornandt L, Kasper W, Bubenheimer P. Reproducibility of Doppler echocardiographic quantification of aortic and mitral valve stenoses: comparison between two echocardiography centers. Am.J.Cardiol. 1991;1991 May 1;67:1013-21.
27. Otto CM, Pearlman AS, Gardner CL, Kraft CD, Fujioka MC. Simplification of the Doppler continuity equation for calculating stenotic aortic valve area. J.Am.Soc.Echocardiogr. 1988;1988 Mar-Apr;1:155-57.
28. Blitz LR, Herrmann HC. Hemodynamic assessment of patients with low-flow, low-gradient valvular aortic stenosis. Am.J.Cardiol. 1996;1996 Sep 15;78:657-61.
29. Burwash IG, Thomas DD, Sadahiro M, Pearlman AS, Verrier ED, Thomas R et al. Dependence of Gorlin formula and continuity equation valve areas on transvalvular volume flow rate in valvular aortic stenosis. Circulation 1994;1994 Feb;89:827-35.
30. Burwash IG, Pearlman AS, Kraft CD, Miyake-Hull C, Healy NL, Otto CM. Flow dependence of measures of aortic stenosis severity during exercise. J.Am.Coll.Cardiol. 1994;1994 Nov 1;24:1342-50.
31. Casale PN, Palacios IF, Abascal VM, Harrell L, Davidoff R, Weyman AE et al. Effects of dobutamine on Gorlin and continuity equation valve areas and valve resistance in valvular aortic stenosis. Am.J.Cardiol. 1992;1992 Nov 1;70:1175-79.
32. De Groff CG, Shandas R, Valdes-Cruz L. Analysis of the effect of flow rate on the Doppler continuity equation for stenotic orifice area calculations: a numerical study. Circulation 1998;1998 Apr 28;97:1597-605.
33. Dumesnil JG, Yoganathan AP. Theoretical and practical differences between the Gorlin formula and the continuity equation for calculating aortic and mitral valve areas [see comments]. Am.J.Cardiol. 1991;1991 Jun 1;67:1268-72.
34. Green GR, Miller DC. Continuing dilemmas concerning aortic valve replacement in patients with advanced left ventricular systolic dysfunction. J.Heart Valve Dis. 1997;1997 Nov;6:562-79.

35. Rask LP, Karp KH, Eriksson NP. Flow dependence of the aortic valve area in patients with aortic stenosis: assessment by application of the continuity equation. J.Am.Soc.Echocardiogr. 1996;1996 May-Jun;9:295-99.

36. Shively BK, Charlton GA, Crawford MH, Chaney RK. Flow dependence of valve area in aortic stenosis: relation to valve morphology. J.Am.Coll.Cardiol. 1998;1998 Mar 1;31:654-60.

37. Faggiano P, Gualeni A, Antonini-Canterin F, Rusconi C, Nicolosi G. Doppler echocardiographic assessment of hemodynamic progression of valvular aortic stenosis over time: comparison between aortic valve resistance and valve area. G.Ital.Cardiol.   1999;1999 Oct;29:1131-36.

38. Ho PP, Pauls GL, Lamberton DF, Portnoff JS, Pai RG, Shah PM. Doppler derived aortic valve resistance in aortic stenosis: its hemodynamic validation. J.Heart Valve Dis. 1994;1994 May;3:283-87.

39. Roger VL, Seward JB, Bailey KR, Oh JK, Mullany CJ. Aortic valve resistance in aortic stenosis: Doppler echocardiographic study and surgical correlation. Am.Heart J. 1997;1997 Nov;134:924-29.

40. Saad RM, Barbetseas J, Olmos L, Rubio N, Zoghbi WA. Application of the continuity equation and valve resistance to the evaluation of St. Jude Medical prosthetic aortic valve dysfunction. Am.J.Cardiol. 1997;1997 Nov 1;80:1239-42.

41. Voelker W, Reul H, Nienhaus G, Stelzer T, Schmitz B, Steegers A et al. Comparison of valvular resistance, stroke work loss, and Gorlin valve area for quantification of aortic stenosis. An in vitro study in a pulsatile aortic flow model. Circulation 1995;1995 Feb 15;91:1196-204.

42. Lee TM, Su SF, Chen MF, Liau CS, Lee YT. Effects of increasing flow rate on aortic stenotic indices: evidence from percutaneous transvenous balloon dilatation of the mitral valve in patients with combined aortic and mitral stenosis [published erratum appears in Heart 1997 Mar; 77(3):294]. Heart 1996;1996 Dec;76:490-94.

43. Ford LE, Feldman T, Chiu YC, Carroll JD. Hemodynamic resistance as a measure of functional impairment in aortic valvular stenosis. Circ.Res. 1990;66:1-7.

44. Lin SS, Roger VL, Pascoe R, Seward JB, Pellikka PA. Dobutamine stress Doppler hemodynamics in patients with aortic stenosis: feasibility, safety, and surgical correlations [see comments]. Am.Heart J. 1998;1998 Dec;136:1010-16.

45. Pop C, Metz D, Tassan-Mangina S, Nazeyrollas P, Jamet B, Maes D et al. [Dobutamine doppler echocardiography in severe aortic stenosis with left ventricular dysfunction. Comparison with postoperative examination] [Apport de l'echocardiographie Doppler sous dobutamine dans le retrecissement aortique serre avec dysfonction ventriculaire gauche. Comparaison aux donnees postoperatoires.]. Arch.Mal Coeur Vaiss. 1999;1999 Nov;92:1487-93.

46. Schwammenthal E, Vered Z, Rabinowitz B, Kaplinsky E, Feinberg MS. Stress echocardiography beyond coronary artery disease. Eur.Heart J. 1997;1997 Jun;18 Suppl D:D130-D137.

47. Takeda S, Rimington H, Chambers J. The relation between transaortic pressure difference and flow during dobutamine stress echocardiography in patients with aortic stenosis. Heart 1999;1999 Jul;82:11-14.

48. Rahimtoola SH. Severe aortic stenosis with low systolic gradient : the good and bad news. [In Process Citation]. Circulation 2000;2000 Apr 25;101:1892-94.

49. Connolly HM, Oh JK, Orszulak TA, Osborn SL, Roger VL, Hodge DO et al. Aortic valve replacement for aortic stenosis with severe left ventricular dysfunction. Prognostic indicators. Circulation 1997;1997 May;%20;95:2395-400.

50. Connolly HM, Oh JK, Schaff HV, Roger VL, Osborn SL, Hodge DO et al. Severe aortic stenosis with low transvalvular gradient and severe left ventricular dysfunction : result of aortic valve replacement in 52 patients. [In Process Citation]. Circulation 2000;2000 Apr 25;101:1940-46.

Section III / Chapter 3

THE ROLE OF TRANSESOPHAGEAL ECHOCARDIOGRAPHY IN THE PERI-OPERATIVE PERIOD

Dr. L.H.B. BAUR

Transesophageal echocardiography has become a commonly used monitor of left ventricular function and of aortic and mitral valve surgery during the last 15 years[1,2]
The success and acceptance of the procedure has frequently been due to the close interaction of the cardiac surgeon and cardiologist and the improved imaging possibilities by multiplane echocardiography. Epicardial echocardiography is now infrequently used and only in those patients in which transesophageal echocardiography is not possible due to oesophageal disease[3]. In all other cases TEE offers more reproducible imaging with less interaction with the surgical field.

AORTIC VALVE DISEASE

Preoperative evaluation
The evolution of aortic valve replacement with mechanical valves to replacement with homografts and xenografts, the Ross procedure and the technique of aortic valve repair has been the driving force for the increasing utility of transesophageal echocardiography (TEE) in the operating room for aortic valve surgery[4]. Pre-operatively, TEE is used to assess the presence and the mechanism of aortic valve regurgitation and the likelihood of reparability[5,6]. Patients with significant fibrosis, thickening or calcification of the valve are usually excluded for valve repair[4]. Those selected for aortic valve repair are patients with aortic regurgitation secondary to congenitally bicuspid aortic valves with prolapse, tricuspid aortic valves with prolapse of one cusp, dilation of the aortic annulus or aortic root and perforation of the aortic cusps due to endocarditis[7]. Aortic valve repair is increasingly used in patients with aortic valve insufficiency due to aortic dissection. In these cases valve frequently valve suspension can be performed successfully[4]. In all these cases, TEE is useful to define the aortic valve structure, the number of leaflets, movement of the cusps, aortic root morphology and the mechanism of aortic regurgitation[8]. Color-flow Doppler can give important information about the origin of the regurgitant jet and the direction of the jet.

The surgeon can than be advised to us the appropriate repair technique. Aortic valve leaflet motion is categorised as normal, restricted, or excessive. Normal leaflet structure and motion, when associated with a significant degree of aortic regurgitation is mostly due to dilation of the aortic root and sinotubular junction[4]. Typically, the regurgitant jet originates centrally and is directed centrally into the left ventricular outflow tract. Valve repair requires a commisuroplasty procedure, with pledged sutures at the commisures to bring the sinotubular ridge inward and allow central coaptation[5].

If aortic regurgitation is identified in the presence of a normal aortic valve, aortic dissection needs to be considered[4.] If aortic dissection is the cause of aortic regurgitation, resuspension of the aortic valve may be feasible. It is than important to determine the size and morphology of the aortic root.

A normal aortic root is characterised by symmetric sinuses and a normal diameter of the sinotubular junction diameter measuring 2 to 3 mm larger than the valvular annular diameter. The normal range of the valvular annular diameter is 19 to 23 mm. Asymmetry with a significant difference between sinotubular diameter and valvular annulus is frequently seen with aortic root pathology.

If aortic dissection is present with normal leaflets and severe aortic regurgitation, preservation of the valve is possible in 70% of cases of type A dissection[10] by resuspension of the aortic valve and insertion of a supracoronary graft to bring the sinotubular ridge inward and allow central coaptation. In these patients, freedom from valve replacement at 10 years is 80-90%[10]. If the valve or aortic root is abnormal, a Bentall procedure is the technique of choice. This is always the procedure of choice in patient with an aortic root greater than 36 mm, aortic annular ectasia, cystic media necrosis or patients with Marfan's syndrome[11]. If the dissection flap extents into the coronary artery ostia, this would necessitate a Carbrol modification of the Bentall procedure. Then, the dissected coronary ostia are isolated as buttons of aortic tissue. This button is then reinforced with a collar of Teflon. Coronary perfusion is re-established with a separate tube graft[12].

Excessive leaflet motion is frequently found in patients with a congenitally bicuspid aortic valve with redundancy and prolapse of the fused cusp. In these cases, a triangular resection of the elongated leaflet can be performed with pledged sutures at the commisures[13]. Aortic valve prolapse in patients with a tricuspid valve involves frequently the right coronary cusp and is due to leaflet fenestration[14]. Again, a triangular resection can be used to equalise the length of the leaflet edges with the opposing leaflet allowing symmetric closure. Imaging of aortic valve prolapse is done with the TEE probe in 120 degrees rotation. Then the direction of the color flow jet determines the site of the prolapse[8].

Degenerative, rheumatic or fibrocalcific aortic valve disease causes aortic regurgitation because of restricted leaflet motion. The mechanism is characterised by thickened leaflets with leaflet coaptation distal to the plane of the annulus and central regurgitation in the presence of a normal size and morphology of the aortic root[4]. Sometimes repair can be done by improving pliability of the aortic valve with débridement or peeling of pannus tissue along planes of dissection[15]. The results are frequently suboptimal due to further damage of the valve[16].

Postoperative evaluation

The success of aortic valve repair can easily assessed by TEE. Typically, a grade 1 aortic valve regurgitation remains after the repair procedure. Even in the case of a perfect result, the valve morphology appears abnormal, because the leaflets may remain thickened, bicuspid or even mildly stenotic. If more than grade 2 aortic insufficiency is present, the mechanism of the insufficiency has to be defined. This to enable the surgeon to determine, if a second repair procedure is possible[13]. If a homograft or stentless xenograft has been implanted or a Ross procedure has been performed, the postoperative TEE examination is necessary to assess postoperative aortic insufficiency and possible complications[17,18,19]. After aortic valve replacement with a homograft or stentless valves, minor degrees of aortic regurgitation may reflect failure to maintain the geometry of the symmetric graft. This can be due to distortion or compression during insertion. Coronary perfusion may be affected by technical difficulties during insertion of the coronary buttons. These more typically involve the right coronary artery with kinking resulting in impairment of flow. One has to consider this complication if new left ventricular wall motion abnormalities are present. Sometimes, it is possible to evaluate proximal flow in the right and left coronary artery with color-flow mapping ad assess flow disturbances. After implantation of a homograft, a stentless xenograft or after a Ross procedure, it is not uncommon to see a echo-free space between the graft and the native aorta[18]. One has to be certain to assure that no flow can be detected in this lumen with color-flow. If flow is present, a loose suture line can be the cause. Bulging of the graft in the aortic lumen can be seen if suture dehiscence or hematoma formation is present[19] If a Ross procedure has been performed, the pulmonic homograft has also to be assessed. In addition to pulmonic insufficiency, narrowing of the distal pulmonary homograft can be present. Postoperative TEE after implantation of a mechanical valve is not needed if the surgeon is certain, that the valve is inserted properly.

MITRAL VALVE DISEASE

Preoperative evaluation

Almost all patients with mitral valve disease are accepted for surgery on the basis of transthoracic or transesophageal echocardiography. Intraoperative TEE has a diagnostic function and can be used to refine the diagnosis and change the operative plan[20] but has also a monitoring function and then used to assess the operative result. During the preoperative examination, the severity and the mechanism of the mitral regurgitation can be determined. One has to take in account, that the severity of the mitral regurgitation can be different from that seen in the ambulatory state due to changes in hemodynamics because of the effects of anaesthesia[21]. The severity of the mitral regurgitation can be assessed by measurement of the regurgitant jet area (REF), measurement of the vena contracta[22] or measurement of the proximal isovelocity surface area (PISA)[23]. Measurement of the regurgitant fraction is difficult in the operating room. Assessment of pulmonary vein flow is useful to distinguish grade 3 and grade 4 mitral insufficiency[24]. It is important to determine the mechanism of mitral valve regurgitation by two dimensional echocardiography combined with color-Doppler imaging. The mechanism can be categorised into excessive, normal or restricted leaflet motion.

Postoperative evaluation

After every mitral valve repair procedure, a transesophageal echocardiogram should be performed to determine if any residual mitral regurgitation is present. If so, the degree and mechanism of postoperative regurgitation has to be determined. Also peri-operative complications, such as left ventricular outflow tract obstruction and systolic anterior movement of the mitral valve have to be assessed[25]. It is important to perform postoperative imaging after the patient has been weaned from bypass and loading conditions, intravascular volume and rhythm have been normalised. If mitral regurgitation more than grade 2 is seen, the patient should return to cardiopulmonary bypass for additional repair or replacement of the valve. Besides mitral valve function, postoperative left ventricular function has to be assessed. Global deterioration of left ventricular function can be a result of occult left ventricular dysfunction before operation, inadequate cardioplegia, ischemia, air embolism[26], volume overload or depressant effects of anaesthetic agents. Infrequently posterior wall ischemia is the result of ligation of the circumflex artery by a suture during placement of the annuplasty ring. Transesophageal echocardiography is not needed after placement of a mechanical or bioprosthetic valve.

DETECTION OF ISCHEMIA

Perioperative monitoring of left ventricular function is particularly important in patients with poor left ventricular function, who undergo a valve repair or replacement combined with myocardial revascularisation[27,28]. New segmental wall motion abnormalities have been shown to occur within seconds after the onset of regional ischemia[29] and is more sensitive than electrocardiographic and hemodynamic monitoring[30]. Echocardiographic evidence of ischemia has a close relation with postoperative outcome[30]. Regional left ventricular function and regional wall motion can be scored with a segmental wall-motion scoring system that is also used for transthoracic echocardiography (table 1). If all wall segments are visible, this scoring system uses the sum of scores of all segments divided by the total number of segments. A wall motion score > 1 is an indication of left ventricular dysfunction. It is important to remember, that myocardial ischemia is not the only cause of regional myocardial dysfunction. Abnormal septal motion can be also be due to right ventricular volume or pressure overload, left bundle branch block, Wolff – Parkinson – White syndrome, right ventricular pacing and severe aortic regurgitation. Although regional wall motion abnormalities occur earlier and are more sensitive for ischemic changes than electrocardiographic ST segment changes, one has to take the high cost into consideration. At this moment, intraoperative ECG monitors frequently incorporate ST-segment analysis, providing a display of ST segment deviation over time. There is as yet no reliable on line regional wall motion tracking system. A problem is also; that regional wall motion abnormalities are frequently due to the phenomenon of stunned and hibernating myocardium, in which mechanical dysfunction is occurring in the absence of impaired coronary perfusion. Therefore, intraoperative echocardiography to monitor ischemia is only appropriate for high-risk patients and for those in whom there are other indications for this technique.

MEASUREMENT OF SYSTOLIC FUNCTION AND PRELOAD

Preload can be defined as the left ventricular volume at end-diastole. Because in the operating room one has not the time to make images in several planes during hemodynamic instability, only short axis images at mid-papillary muscle are monitored and the enddiastolic is considered a substitute for preload and enddiastolic volume. Simultaneous measurement of enddiastolic and endsystolic areas with radionuclide angiography showed correlations between 0.85 and 0.92 for volumes and a correlation of 0.96 for ejection fraction[2,31]. The correlation of left ventricular enddiastolic area with conventional measures of preload such as pulmonary artery diastolic pressure or pulmonary capillary wedge pressure appeared to be disappointing[32,33]. In the diagnosis of postoperative hypovolemia, when systemic hypotension is accompanied by high filling pressures TEE appears to be more sensitive than measurement of central venous pressure or pulmonary artery pressure[34]. To improve on-line tracking of left ventricular size and function, automatic border detection has been developed. The algorithm relies on the different acoustic properties of tissue and fluid, which permit the display of endocardial borders. The drawback of this system is that the frequently occurring dropout in the lateral portions of the image leads to frequent inaccuracies. Various investigators have reported success with ABD in only 56 to 78% of cases because of inadequacies of images[35,36] Comparison of ABD with radionuclide methods and ultrafast computed tomography showed, that ABD tended to underestimate end-diastolic areas and ejection fraction and overestimate endsystolic area[35,37]. Intraoperative echocardiography is also used to help position intracardiac catheters, including those used for retrograde cardioplegia via the coronary sinus[38].

Table 1. Segmental Wall-Motion Scoring System

Score	Wall Motion	Radial Shortening	Myocardial Thickening
1	Normal	> 30%	+++
2	Hypokinesia	0 – 30 %	++
3	Akinesia	0	0
4	Dyskinesia	Systolic lengthening	Systolic thinning

REFERENCES

1. Sheikh KH, de Bruijn NP, Rankin JS, Clements FM, Stanley T, Wolfe WG, Kisslo J. The utility of transesophageal echocardiography and Doppler color flow imaging in patients undergoing cardiac valve surgery. J Am Coll Cardiol 15:363-372;1990.
2. Urbanowitz J, Shaabon J, Cohen N, Cahalau MK, Botvinick EH, Chatterjee K, Schiller NB, Dae MW, Matthay MA. Comparison of transesophageal echocardiographic and scintigrapic estimates of left ventricular end-diastolic volume index and ejection fraction in patients following coronary artery bypass grafting. Anesthesiology 1990;72:607-612.
3. Stewart WJ, Thomas JT, Klein AL: Ten year trends in utilization of 6340 intraoperative echocardiograms. Circulation 92:SI-514,1995.
4. Grimm RA, Stewart WJ. The Role of intraoperative echocardiography in valve surgery. Cardiology Clinics 16: 477-489; 1998.
5. Cosgrove DM, Rosenkrantz ER, Hendren WG, Bartlett JC, Stewart WJ. Valvuloplasty for aortic insufficiency. J. Thorac. Cardiovasc. Surg. 102: 571-576; 1991
6. Underwood MJ, Khoury GE, Deronck D, Glineur D, Dion R. The aortic root: structure, function, and surgical reconstruction. Heart 2000; 83: 376-380.
7. Stewart WJ: Intraoperative echocardiography. In Skorton D (ed): Cardiac Imaging-Principles and Practice. Philadelphia, WB Saunders, 1996, 566-581.
8. Cohen GI, Duffy CI, Klein AL, Miller DP, Cosgrove DM, Stewart WJ. Color Doppler and two-dimensional echocardiographic determination of the mechanism of aortic regurgitation with surgical correlation. J. Am. Soc. Echocardiogr. 9: 508-515; 1996.
9. Mazzucotelli JP, Deleuze PH, Baufreton C, Duval AM, Hillion ML, Loisance DY, Cachera JP. Preservation of the aortic valve in acute aortic dissection: Long-term echocardiographic assessment and clinical outcome. Ann. Thorac. Surg. 55: 1513,1993.
10. Glower DD, Speier RA, White WD, Smith LR, Rankin JS, Wolfe WG. Management and long-term outcome of aortic dissection. Ann. Surg. 214: 31-41, 1991.
11. Griepp R: Glenn's thoracic and cardiovascular surgery. In Baue AE (ed): Dissections of the aorta. Stmford, CT, Appleton & Lange, 1996, 2285-2298.
12. Cabrol C, Pavie A, Meznildray P, Gandjbakhchi I, Langhlink, Bors V, Coros T. Long-term results with total replacement of the ascending aorta and re-implantation of the coronary arteries. J. Thorac. Cardiovasc. Surg. 8: 678 -692,1993.
13. Fraser C, Wang N, Mee RB, Lytle BW, McCarthy PM, Sapp SK, Rozenkranz ER, Cosgrove BM. Repair of insufficient bicuspid aortic valves. Ann. Thorac. Surg. 58: 386-390, 1994.
14. Tatsuno K, Konno S, Ando M, Sahakibara S. Pathogenic mechanisms of prolapsing aortic valve and aortic regurgitation associated with ventricular septal defect. Circulation 48: 1028-1037; 1973.
15. Duran C, Kumar N, Gometza B, Al Halees Z. Indications and limitations of aortic valve reconstruction. Ann. Thorac. Surg. 52: 447-453, 1991.
16. Duran CM, Gometza B Aortic valve reconstruction in the young. J. Cardiovasc. Surg. 9: 204-208, 1994.
17. Petrou M, Wong K, Albertucci M, Yacoub MH. Evaluation of unstented aortic homografts for the treatment of prosthetic aortic valve endocarditis. Circulation 90: II-198- II-204, 1994.
18. Baur LHB, Kappetein AP, Peels CA, van der Ploeg A, Sieders A, Bootsma M, van Wely M, Hazekamp M, van der Wall EE, Huysmans HA. Echocardiographic imaging of the Freestyle® stentless aortic valve prosthesis. Echocardiography in press.
19. Van Roosmalen R, Baur LHB, Braun J, Atsma D, Hazekamp M, van der Wall EE, Huysmans HA. Dynamic Obstruction, an unusual complication of stentless bioprostheses. Int. J. Cardiac Imaging 15; 209-214, 1999.
20. Secknus MA, Klein AL, Smedira NG, *** Does pre pump operative echocardiography change operative plans in mitral valve repair? J. Am. Soc. Echocardiogr. 9: 374-***,1996.

21. Nishimura RA, Abel MD, Housmans PR, Warnes CA, Tajik AJ. Mitral flow velocity curves as a function of different loading conditions: Evaluation by intraoperative transesophageal Doppler echocardiography. J. Am. Soc. Echocardiogr. 2: 79-87, 1989.

22. Tribouilloy C, Shen WF, Quere JP, Rey JL, Choquet D, Dufosse D, Dufosse H, Leslie JP Assessment of severity of mitral regurgitation by measuring regurgitant jet width at its origin with transesophageal Doppler color flow imaging. Circulation 85: 1248-1253, 1992.

23. Rivera JM, Vandervoort PM, Thoreau DH, Levine RA, Weyman AE, Thomas JD Quantification of mitral regurgitation using the proximal flow method: A clinical study. Am. Heart J. 124: 1289-1296, 1992.

24. Klein AL, Obarski TP, Stewart WJ, Casale PN, Paerce GL, Husbands K, Cosgrove DM, Salcedo EE Transesophageal Doppler echocardiography of pulmonary venous flow: A new marker of mitral regurgitation severity. J. Am. Coll. Cardiol. 18:518-526,1991.

25. Stewart WJ, Salcedo EE, Cosgrove DM. The value of echocardiography in mitral valve repair. Clev. Clin. J. Med. 58: 177-183, 1991.

26. Rodigas P, Meyer FS, Haasler GB, Dubroff JM, Spotnitz HM Intra-operative two-dimensional echocardiography: Ejection of microbubbles from the left ventricle after cardiac surgery. Am. J. Cardiol. 50: 1130-1132, 1982.

27. Topol EJ, Weiss JL, Guzman PA, Dorsey-Lima S, Blanck TJ, Humphrey LS, Baumgartner WA, Flakerty TJ, Reitz BA Immediate improvement of dysfunctional myocardial segments after coronary revascularization: Detection by intraoperative transesophageal echocardiography. J. Am. Coll. Cardiol. 1984; 4: 1123-1134.

28. Lazar HL, Plehn JF, Schick EM, Dobnick D, Shemin RJ Effects of coronary revascularization on regional wall motion. J. Thorac. Cardiovasc. Surg. 1989; 98: 498-505.

29. Vatner SF: Correlation between acute reductions in myocardial blood flow and function in conscious dogs. Circ. Res. 47: 201-207, 1980.

30. Leung JM, O' Kelly B, Browner WS, Tubau J, Hollenberg M, Manjano DT Prognostic importance of postbypass wall motion abnormalities in patients undergoing coronary artery bypass graft surgery. Anesthesiology 1989; 71: 16-25.

31. Clements FM, Harpole DH, Quill T, Jones RH. McCann RL. Estimation of left ventricular volume and ejection fraction by two-dimensional transesophageal echocardiography : comparison of short axis imaging and simultaneous radionuclide angiography. Br. J.Anaesth. 1990;64:331-336.

32. Hansen RH, Viquerat CE, Matthay MA, Wiener-Kronish JP, De Marco T, Baktia S, Marks J, Botvinick EH, Chatterjee K Poor correlation between pulmonary arterial wedge pressure and left ventricular end-diastolic volume after coronary artery bypass graft surgery. Anesthesiology 1986; 64: 764-770.

33. Thys DM, Hillel Z, Goldman ME, Mindick BP, Kaplan JA A comparison of hemodynamic indices derived by invasive monitoring and two-dimensional echocardiography. Anesthesiology 1987; 67: 630-634.

34. Leung JM. Levine EH. Left ventricular end-systolic cavity obliteration as an estimate of intraoperative hypovolemia. Anesthesiology. 1994; 81:1102-1109.

35. Marcus RH, Bednarz J, Coulden R, Shroff S. Lipton M. Lang RM Ultrasonic backscatter system for automated on-line endocardial border detection: Evaluation by ultrafast computed tomography. J. Am. Coll. Cardiol. 1993; 22: 839-847.

36. Cahalan MK, Ionescu P, Melton H Jr, Adler S, Keel L, Schiller NB Automated real-time analysis of intraoperative transesophageal echocardiograms. Anestesiology 1993; 78: 477-485.

37. Gorcsan J, Lazar JM, Schulman DS, Follansbee WP Comparison of left ventricular function by echocardiographic automated border detection and radionuclide ejection farction. Am. J. Cardiol. 1993; 72; 810-815.
38. Orihashi K, Hong YW, Chung G, Sioto D, Goldiner PL, Oka Y: New applications of two-dimensional transesophageal echocardiography in cardiac surgery. J. Cardiothor. Vasc. Anesth. 1991; 5: 33-39.

Section III / Chapter 4

EVALUATION OF VALVE DISEASE WITH NOVEL IMAGING TECHNIQUES

Prof.Dr. E.E. VAN DER WALL

INTRODUCTION

Of the novel imaging techniques for detection of valve disease, magnetic resonance (MR) imaging has made the most relevant progress over the past years. Newest advances in MR technology allow for highly accurate measurements of left atrial and ventricular dimensions, and regurgitant volumes. Therefore, MR techniques may become the first method of choice for quantitative evaluation of regurgitant valves. For assessment of valve stenosis severity, measurement of transvalvular pressure gradient is an appropriate measure. MR imaging may not be advantageous over echocardiography, provided the ultrasound window is adequate. With respect to surgical treatment, valvular morphology is of major importance, and in this setting echocardiography still appears to be the first line method. Little information is available on the relation valve lesion severity and/or morphology to clinical outcome. Conversely, the extent of cardiac adaptation to pressure overload and/or volume overload, i.e. ventricular remodeling, is a major predictor of outcome, and is therefore most relevant for final patient judgement. For assessment of left and right ventricular remodeling, echocardiography typically provides all the necessary information. However, in special cases with discrepant findings, with inadequate ultrasound window, or in the preoperative work-up, MR imaging may provide important information regarding cardiac adaptation to valvular lesions. In addition, flow velocity mapping provides reliable estimations of valve gradients and flows across valves.

TECHNICAL ASPECTS IN MR IMAGING

For a better understanding of valve morphology and function some of the most relevant technical aspects are discussed. The most prominent characteristics of MR imaging are its high soft tissue contrast without the need for contrast medium application and the capability to quantify blood flow using flow-velocity mapping.

Flow-velocity mapping is based on the fact that the phase shift of the MR signal of blood flowing along a magnetic field gradient is proportional to the blood flow velocity. Both flow velocities and flow volumes can be reliably measured. Several imaging strategies have been developed to decrease the effect of cardiac motion. To resolve highly pulsatile flow patterns appropriate temporal resolution is needed.

High spatial resolution is required not only to depict thin anatomic structures such as the heart valves but also to reduce intravoxel dephasing when encoding velocities in complex flow fields. In order to compensate for cardiac motion, prospective or retrospective ECG triggering is usually applied. Recently, real time MR imaging [12, 36, 62] has become available that acquires images in as fast as 15 ms thereby freezing cardiac motion. Correction of respiratory motion typically involves either breath holding approaches or alternatively, correction algorithms allowing data acquisition during free breathing. Breath-holding is in general a robust method to eliminate respiratory motion as long as patient co-operation is obtained. Its major limitations include rather low temporal resolution since segmented k space strategies are typically required to shorten acquisition time. Furthermore, exact localisation of the imaging plane is uncertain as long as heart position is not monitored during breath holding. On the other hand, free breathing approaches allow for excellent temporal resolution since minimal constraints exist with respect to imaging time. One major limitation arises from the fact that diaphragmatic motion monitored by navigator imaging does not always reflect cardiac motion accurately. Future solutions may employ several navigators placed directly on the heart surfaces. Third-generation scanners use almost real-time, multislice 3-D imaging features without the need for breathholding.

CONTRAINDICATIONS TO MR IMAGING

Pacemakers, cochlear implants and electronical devices (pacemakers, automatic implantable cardioverters) are contraindicated to undergo MR studies. Claustrophobia (2-5% of cases) may be a limiting factor, particularly for longer studies. In general, atrial fibrillation severely degrades image quality and variable length of diastole further affects accuracy of hemodynamic measurements. The use of real-time approaches may avoid the limitations inherent to severe rhythm disturbances.

AORTIC VALVE STENOSIS

In patients with aortic valve stenosis concentric left ventricular hypertrophy is the main adaptation mechanism to reduce left ventricular systolic wall stress. During early stages of the disease ejection fraction is preserved [44, 54]. An aortic valve area below 0.75 cm^2 is usually considered severe aortic valve stenosis. When cardiac output is normal and aortic valve stenosis is severe, the mean transvalvular pressure gradient is high. Doppler echocardiography is typically used to measure transvalvular pressure gradients. A similar approach has been adopted for MR assessment of aortic valve stenosis [11,22,51]. In patients with moderate to severe aortic valve stenosis agreement between echocardiographically and MR-imaging derived mean pressure gradients is excellent. Also Kilner et al.[22] showed this phenomenon both for aortic valve stenosis and mitral valve stenosis, where average peak velocity of 4 pixels was assumed to represent peak velocity. For both echocardiography and MR imaging, flow velocity mapping has to be applied parallel to the velocity jet in order to capture peak valve velocities. In patients with suboptimal ultrasound window, MR imaging may be used as an alternative since no limitations with respect to imaging plane angle exist. Patients with severe aortic valve stenosis and low cardiac output frequently present with relatively low pressure gradients [16]. Separation of these patients from those with mild to moderate aortic valve stenosis may be difficult. It is therefore recommended to include a cardiac output measurement in an MR study for aortic valve stenosis assessment.

Progression of lesion severity is rather low in aortic valve stenosis patients and more than 50% of the reported patients showed little progression over three to 9 years [59]. Therefore, in patients with severe aortic valve stenosis, the ACC/AHA guidelines recommend annual echocardiographic or MR imaging studies for monitoring valve gradients and left ventricular function [1]. In symptomatic patients with severe aortic valve stenosis, aortic valve replacement is indicated, since average survival after onset of symptoms is less than 2 to 3 years [20,59]. Postoperative mortality due to the valve prosthesis occurs at a relatively low rate of approximately 1% per year [17]. Several clinical studies reported asymptomatic patients with severe aortic valve stenosis at particularly high risk for complications and death, justifying aortic valve replacement even in the absence of symptoms in these patients [29]. Myocardial fibrosis associated with left ventricular hypertrophy may preclude complete functional recovery and hence, aortic valve replacement in a-symptomatic patients with severe aortic valve stenosis and reduced left ventricular function or excessive left ventricular hypertrophy may be considered as a relative indication. Since MR imaging is ideally suited in assessing left ventricular function and left ventricular hypertrophy [28,41,43] it may provide the necessary information to identify high-risk patients with aortic valve stenosis.

AORTIC VALVE INSUFFICIENCY

In patients with chronic aortic valve regurgitation left ventricular remodeling allows recruitment of preload reserve and thereby maintains normal contractile performance despite elevated afterload [39]. While these mechanisms are operative in the compensated stage, the balance between afterload excess, preload reserve and hypertrophy cannot be preserved indefinitely. With progression of disease further increase in afterload may result in reduction of left ventricular ejection fraction [39].

At this stage increased filling pressures may cause dyspnea and an impaired flow reserve of hypertrophied myocardium may result in angina pectoris [34].

It is during this transition from compensated to decompensated volume overload hypertrophy, where patients might undergo aortic valve replacement [5,14,23,30]. In aortic regurgitation patients, the mortality rate in patients with angina exceeds 10% per year, and in patients with heart failure it is higher than 20% per year [18,37]. In addition, more than 25% of patients with aortic regurgitation die or develop left ventricular dysfunction before the onset of warning symptoms [4, 45,46,50]. There is general agreement that symptomatic patients should undergo aortic valve replacement[1]. Patients should be monitored noninvasively over time. Aortic valve replacement is indicated when left ventricular ejection fraction does not increase during exercise or left ventricular chamber dilatation is substantial (enddiastolic diameter >75 mm or endsystolic diameter >55 mm). Since assessment of left ventricular function plays a central role in the management of a-symptomatic aortic valve regurgitation, the echocardiographically determined left ventricular function has to be confirmed by an additional measurement, such as a second echocardiogram, a radionuclide angiogram, or an MR imaging study [1, 57]. A large number of echocardiographic studies are available with respect to prognostic significance of left ventricular dimensions and other geometrical parameters for postoperative outcome [9,14,23]. Although MR imaging has been shown to be highly accurate in determining left ventricular function and volumes [28, 41], it has not been used to define criteria predicting postoperative left ventricular function or clinical outcome. The potential of MR imaging in assessing left ventricular function has also recently been shown in a study of patients with aortic regurgitation [15].

Assessment of the severity of aortic regurgitation by echocardiography is based on Doppler measurements of color flow jet area and color flow width. Indirect measures of regurgitant volume are the rate of decline in regurgitant gradient defined by the pressure half time and the presence of flow reversal in the descending aorta. [8,26,56]. In addition, comparison of stroke volume of pulmonary or mitral valves with that of the aortic valve may provide a quantitative measure of valvular lesion severity [61]. In patients with poor ultrasound windows, equivocal findings, and controversial data results such as in patients with mild regurgitation and severe left ventricular dysfunction, MR imaging may be considered as the method of choice for further evaluation [57]. By means of flow-velocity mapping through the aortic root, anterograde and retrograde blood flow during the cardiac cycle is quantified and provides accurate measures of regurgitant volume and regurgitant fraction [10, 19, 38, 52]. Walker et al. [60] suggested a control volume approach for quantification of regurgitant volumes similar to the proximal isovelocity surface area method. This elegant method has been shown to accurately quantify regurgitant volumes in vitro. Several limitations may arise from the need for adjustment of the position of the control volume during the cardiac cycle with respect to the position of the aortic valve. A practically more feasible approach has recently been suggested by Kozerke et al. [25]. Using this approach the plane of velocity encoding is moving with the aortic valve during the cardiac cycle. Currently, this technique is incorporated in a clinical protocol that lasts approximately 1 hour and provides measures of regurgitant volume, stroke volume, cardiac output, left ventricular enddiastolic and endsystolic volumes, ejection fraction, and left ventricular mass.

In addition to the detection of aortic valve lesions, pathology of the aortic root has to be described. MR imaging is an accurate method for evaluation of the aortic root [55].

Patients with dilatation of the aortic root exceeding 50 mm should undergo reconstructive surgery combined with aortic valve replacement [27].

MITRAL VALVE STENOSIS

In addition to the assessment of symptoms, the essential issues of the diagnostic work-up of a patient with mitral valve stenosis are the hemodynamic assessment of mitral stenosis severity, the morphological assessment of the mitral valve apparatus, and the assessment of pulmonary hypertension. Generally, rheumatic heart disease is the major cause of patients with mitral stenosis. Approximately 40% of these patients present with isolated valve stenosis [40]. With the advent of percutaneous mitral balloon valvulotomy, a technique is available with immediate [31] and long-term [3] similar to those of open commissurotomy. Since percutaneous mitral balloon valvulotomy is the treatment of choice in patients with mitral valve stenosis[1], assessment of mitral valve suitability for percutaneous valvulotomy is of major importance in the management of mitral stenosis patients, particularly in patients with mild symptoms. Since 2-D echocardiography and Doppler echocardiography provide the necessary information to monitor most patients with mitral valve stenosis, there is generally no need for additional MR imaging studies. In patients with a discrepancy between symptoms and hemodynamics, an MR imaging study may add confirmatory data regarding the severity of the transvalvular pressure gradients [22]. For patients with severe mitral stenosis and grade 3 or 4 mitral regurgitation, percutaneous balloon valvulotomy is contraindicated and flow-velocity based quantification of regurgitation may identify patients who should undergo open commissurotomy.

MITRAL VALVE REGURGITATION

In patients with severe non-ischemic mitral regurgitation the mitral valve prolapse syndrome is usually the most common cause. In a large series form the Mayo Clinics [58], including 478 patients with severe mitral regurgitation (approximately 80% with mitral valve prolapse syndrome), preoperative NYHA Class I/II was associated with an excellent prognosis after mitral valve surgery (84% mitral valve repair). Expected survival was not different from observed survival in these patients and it was concluded that surgery of severe organic mitral valve regurgitation should be considered even in patients with no or minimal symptoms. The surgical method of choice is mitral valve repair, since its operative risk is low (0.5% for all ages, and 0% for patients <75 years [2]. In case mitral valve surgery is recommended before symptoms develop, left ventricular dilatation and left ventricular dysfunction may occur as indirect markers of severe volume overload and, direct quantification of regurgitation fraction or regurgitant volume would become crucial for patient management. Recently, an elegant method for quantification of mitral regurgitation by flow velocity mapping was presented by Fujita et al. [13]. Mitral regurgitation was calculated as left ventricular inflow through the mitral valve minus left ventricular outflow in the ascending aorta. "Regurgitant volume" of healthy volunteers closely approached zero and patients with mild, moderate, and severe mitral regurgitation as assessed by Doppler criteria were clearly separated by flow-velocity mapping. One major limitation of that study was the cyclic motion of the mitral annulus relative to the imaging plane during the cardiac cycle which was not corrected for. Currently, we are using a modification of this approach [63]. Similar to the procedure presented for aortic regurgitation quantification, displacement data of the base of the heart are used to adjust the plane of velocity encoding for diastolic mitral valve motion. This approach is also applicable in patients with aortic valve regurgitation, since diastolic left ventricular inflow (defined as left ventricular mitral inflow and aortic regurgitation volume) is equal to the systolic left ventricular outflow (defined as aortic outflow and mitral regurgitant volume). An alternative to flow-velocity mapping in case of absent aortic regurgitation is to measure enddiastolic and endsystolic right and left ventricular volumes for quantification of right and left ventricular inflow [28] and thus, regurgitant volume [47]. The control volume approach was recently validated in vitro for the mitral valve [7]. Although conceptually attractive, this approach is rather time-consuming (> 1 hour acquisition time for 3-D velocity data of the control volume) and difficulty in correcting the position of the control volume for the cyclic motion of the mitral valve may further limit its practical applicability.

For a comprehensive assessment of patients with mitral valve regurgitation, several parameters should be established such as quantification of regurgitation, assessment of left ventricular adaptation to volume-overload, and anatomy of mitral valve and subvalvular apparatus. Whereas MR imaging meets the first two issues, echocardiography remains the method of choice for assessment of valve anatomy. Although improvements in MR imaging strategies allow detection of morphological abnormalities such as flail mitral valve leaflets, the ability of echocardiography to scan the mitral valve in multiple views in a very short time provides considerable advantages over MR imaging at the present time. The evaluation of patients with mitral regurgitation should therefore begin with echocardiography to determine mitral valve morphology and to provide a grading of valve regurgitation severity. In a next phase, severity of mitral regurgitation is quantified/confirmed by MR imaging. This approach would yield a quantitative measure of mitral regurgitation (e.g. regurgitant volume/m^2 body surface area) enabling estimation of the maximum possible relief of volume-overload in a given patient. According to the guidelines of the ACC/AHA, serial testing is aimed to assess changes in symptoms and to objectively assess changes in left ventricular function and exercise tolerance [1]. If accurate quantification of mitral valve regurgitation becomes available by means of flow-velocity mapping, such information may be useful in monitoring patients with mild to moderate valve regurgitation and may help identifying patients in the phase of transition from moderate to severe mitral regurgitation.

Generally accepted indications for mitral valve surgery are severe mitral regurgitation in symptomatic patients, and in asymptomatic or mildly symptomatic patients with left ventricular dysfunction (ejection fraction$\leq$ 40%) and /or left ventricular dilatation (endsystolic diameter $\geq$45 mm) [1]. In patients with suboptimal echocardiographic windows. MR imaging is an alternative for the evaluation of the hemodynamic consequences of severe mitral valve regurgitation providing information of regurgitant volume, left ventricular dimensions and left ventricular function [57].

In patients with ischemic mitral regurgitation, prognosis is considerably worse than that of other causes of mitral regurgitation [2]. Assessment of ischemia of the posterior wall and the papillary muscles, respectively, is crucial in these patients. MR imaging may provide information regarding myocardial ischemia by means of dobutamine MR stress imaging [33] or direct MR perfusion imaging [42].

TRICUSPID VALVE DISEASE

In principal, the MR imaging approaches to assess mitral and aortic valve disease are also applicable to the tricuspid and pulmonary valves. Kayser et al. [21] showed the importance of tricuspid annular motion correction when measuring tricuspid flow. This correction was achieved by subtracting velocities measured in soft tissue surrounding the valve from the registered velocities through the tricuspid valve. The authors presented normal and pathological values characterizing right ventricular inflow [21]. A tagging approach as mentioned for the mitral and aortic valve is also applicable to correct for cyclic motion of the right-sided base of the heart.

PULMONIC VALVE DISEASE

The vast majority of pulmonary valve lesions are congenital in origin and echocardiographic assessment is straightforward. The Natural History Study data [32, 35] suggest that mild pulmonary valve stenosis is a benign disease and that moderate/severe pulmonary valve stenosis should undergo either balloon valvulotomy or surgery, which both provide excellent prognosis with a low rate of recurrence. Due to the irregular shape of the right ventricle, echocardiography as well as right ventricular angiography are limited in accurate measurements of volumes and muscle mass. MR has been repeatedly demonstrated to provide highly reproducible data on right ventricular volumes and mass [28,47]. In patients with discrepancies between pulmonary stenosis severity and clinical symptoms, MR imaging may be added to allow for quantification of right ventricular dimensions and function [57]. Pulmonary regurgitation may occur after successful repair of Fallot's tetralogy. In this patient population, a comprehensive assessment of pulmonary regurgitation severity, right ventricular remodeling, and pathology of pulmonary circulation may be obtained by an MR study including anatomical and functional assessment of pulmonary circulation by MR angiography and flow measurements.

MIXED VALVULAR DISEASE

In patients with complicated valvular lesions such as mitral valve stenosis and regurgitation in combination with aortic valve stenosis and regurgitation, it is theoretically possible to quantify each lesion using MR techniques. This can be done by measuring left ventricular inflow through the mitral valve, left ventricular outflow through the aortic valve, and regurgitant aortic volume. Flow quantification by MR imaging depends on the assumption of uniform velocity distribution within each voxel and phase alterations due to turbulence may limit the accuracy of flow measurements. Accordingly, in combined aortic valve stenosis and regurgitation the preferred measurements site of total left ventricular systolic outflow is the left ventricular outflow tract to avoid regions of major turbulence. In patients with a mixed single valve lesion, the additional measurement of left ventricular stroke volume from anatomical volumetric data sets may allow for an objective assessment of the quality of the MR imaging data. In patients with combined aortic regurgitation/aortic stenosis and an intact mitral valve, total left ventricular outflow through the aortic valve measured by flow-velocity mapping is expected to be equal to total left ventricular stroke volume measured volumetrically by MR imaging. Since Doppler-based continuity equation calculation of valve area may not be completely independent of flow [6], and invasive determination of cardiac volumes may be difficult in very large and/or spherical left ventricles [48], an additional MR study may be useful in complicated settings of mixed valvular disease. This holds particularly for patients with impaired left ventricular function in which double versus single valve surgery would bear a substantially increased risk. Measurement of total left ventricular outflow by flow-velocity mapping and accurate quantification of left ventricular hypertrophy may add integrative information for clinical decision making.

The combination of mitral valve stenosis and aortic regurgitation may present diagnostic difficulties particularly with regard to assessment of severity of aortic regurgitation severity in patients with severe mitral stenosis. Mitral valve stenosis restricts left ventricular filling, thereby blunting the impact of aortic regurgitation on left ventricular dilatation. Flow-based quantification of aortic regurgitation may help resolving diagnostic problems.

PROSTHETIC VALVES

Mechanical valves, except the outdated Starr-Edwards valve, are safe in the MR environment since the materials are not ferromagnetic [49,53]. However, mechanical valves are prone to artifacts that prevent a direct visualization of the device.

Recently, the unique ability of MR techniques to encode velocities with high temporal and spatial resolution was exploited to describe the flow field distal to mechanical heart valves in patients. Such applications are potentially useful to verify model calculations in-vivo and should allow for improving designs of mechanical valves. Most valves are mounted on rigid or flexible stents that may cause artifacts.

Assessment of bioprostheses by MR imaging is fortunately not hampered by artifacts.

CONCLUSIONS

The most relevant issues in the assessment of patients with valvular heart disease are the detection of valve lesion severity, the morphological description of heart valve and subvalvular structures, and the assessment of changes of the ventricles and the pulmonary circulation. MR imaging is an excellent, accurate and reproducible tool for the assessment of valve lesion severity and to monitor cardiac adaptation to volume and/or pressure-overload. An excellent overview of MR imaging in valvular disease is given by Schwitter [42]. Due to the unique capability of MR techniques to measure flow, MR flow-velocity mapping may be particularly useful in quantification of regurgitant lesions and also in the serial assessment of changes of the heart. In the determination of stenotic lesion severity, MR imaging offers no direct advantages over echocardiography provided that echocardiographic window is adequate. Generally, 2-D echocardiography is the first method of choice in the assessment of valve lesion severity. Currently, MR techniques are generally accepted as a highly accurate technique for noninvasive measurement of blood flow, quantification of chamber dimensions, and assessment of ventricular function. With MR imaging it is possible to acquire data of lesion severity, left ventricular dimensions, and left ventricular function within 1 hour or less. In the near future, real time imaging capabilities will become routine and will shorten MR studies substantially. Consequently, there is a growing potential for application of MR imaging in patients with suspected or known valvular heart disease.

REFERENCES

1. ACC/AHA guidelines for the management of patients with valvular heart disease. A report of the American College of Cardiology/American Heart Association. Task Force on Practice Guidelines (Committee on Management of Patients with Valvular Heart Disease). J Am Coll Cardiol 1998;32:1486-588.

2. Akins CW, Hilgenberg AD, Buckley MJ, et al. Mitral valve reconstruction versus replacement for degenerative or ischemic mitral regurgitation. Ann Thorac Surg 1994;58:668-75.

3. Ben Farhat M, Ayari M, Maatouk F, et al. Percutaneous balloon versus surgical closed and open mitral commissurotomy: seven-year follow-up results of a randomized trial. Circulation 1998;97:245-50.

4. Bonow RO, Lakatos E, Maron BJ, et al. Serial long-term assessment of the natural history of a-symptomatic patients with chronic aortic regurgitation and normal left ventricular systolic function. Circulation 1991;84:1625-35.

5. Borer JS, Hochreiter C, Herrold EM, et al. Prediction of indications for valve rreplacement among a-symptomatic or minimally symptomatic patients with chronic aortic regurgitation and normal left ventricular performance. Circulation 1998:97:525-34.

6. Burwash IG, Thomas DD, Sadahir M, et al. Dependence of Gorlin formula and continuity equation valve areas on transvalvular volume flow rate in valvular aortic stenosis. Circulation 1994;89:827-35.

7. Chatzimavroudis GP, Oshinski JN, Pettigrew RI, et al. Quantification of mitral regurgitation with MR phase-velocity mapping using a control volume method. J Magn Reson Imaging 1998:8:577-82.

8. Cheitlin MD, Alpert JS, Armstrong WF, et al. ACC/AHA guidelines for the clinical application of echocardiography. Circulation 1997;95:1686-744.

9. Daniel WG, Hood WJ, Siart A, et al. Chronic aortic regurgitation: reassessment of the prognostic value of preoperative left ventricular end-systolic dimension and fractional shortening. Circulation 1985;71:669-80.

10. Dulce MC, Mostbeck GH, O'Sullivan M, et al. Severity of aortic regurgitation: interstudy reproducibility of measurements with velocity-encoded cine MR imaging. Radiology 1992;185:235-40.

11. Eichenberger AC, Jenni R, von Schulthess GK. Aortic valve pressure gradients in patients with aortic valve stenosis: quantification with velocity-encoded cine MR imaging. Am J Roentgenol 1993;160:971-7.

12. Eichenberger AC, Schwitter J, McKinnon GC, et al. Phase-contrast echo-planar MR imaging: real-time guantification of flow and velocity patterns in the thoracic vessels induced by Valsalva's maneuver. J Magn Reson Imaging 1995;5:648-55.

13. Fujita N, Chazouilleres AF, Hartiala JJ, et al. Quantification of mitral regurgitation by velocity-encoded cine nuclear magnetic resonance imaging. J Am Coll Cardiol 1994;23:951-8.

14. Gaasch WH, Carroll JD, Levine HJ, et al. Chronic aortic regurgitation: prognostic value of left ventricular end-systolic dimension and end-diastolic radius/thickness ratio. J Am Coll Cardiol 19883;1:775-82.

15. Globits S, Blake L, Bourne M, et al. Assessment of hemodynamic effects of angiotensin-converting enzyme inhibitor therapy in chronic aortic regurgitation by using velocity-encoded cine magnetic resonance imaging. Am Heart J 1996;131:289-93.

16. Gorlin R, Gorlin SG. Hydraulic formula for calculation of the area of stenotic mitral valve,other cardiac valvues and central circulatory shunts. Am Heart 1951;41:1-29.

17. Hammermeister KE, Sethi GK, Henderson WG, et al. A comparison of outcomes in men 11 years after heart-valve replacement with a mechanical valve or bioprosthesis. Veterans Affairs Cooperative Study on Valvular Heart Disease. N Engl J Med 1993;328:1289-96.

18. Hegglin R, Scheu H, Rothlin M. Aortic insufficiency. Circulation 1968;38:77-92.

19. Honda N, Machida K, Hashimoto M, et al. Aortic regurgitation: quantitation with MR imaging velocity mapping. Radiology 1993;186:189-94.
20. Livanainen AM, Lindroos M, Tilvis R, et al. Natural history of aortic valve stenosis of varying severity in the elderly. Am J Cardiol 1996;78:97-101.
21. Kayser HW, Stoel BC, van der Wall E, et al. MR velocity mapping of tricuspid flow: correction for through-plane motion. J Magn Reson Imaging 1997;7:669-73.
22. Kilner PJ, Manzara CC, Mohiaddin RH, et al. Magnetic resonance jet velocity mapping in mitral and aortic valve stenosis. Circulation 1993;87:1239-48.
23. Klodas E, Enrique SM, Tajik AJ, et al. Aortic regurgitation complicated by extreme left ventricular dilation: long-term outcome after surgical correction. J Am Coll Cardiol 1996;27:670-7.
24. Kozerke S, Hasenkam JM, Pedersen EM, et al. Particle trace visualization of flow patterns downstream of a prosthetic aortic valve in patients. 7th Scientific Meeting of the ISMRM, Philadelphia 1999;3:2026.
25. Kozerke S, Scheidegger MB, Pederson EM, et al. Heart motion adapted cine phase-contrast flow measurements through the aortic valve. Magn Reson Med 1999;42:970-8.
26. Labovitz AJ, Ferrera RP, Kern MJ, et al. Quantitative evaluation of aortic insufficiency by continuous wave Doppler echocardiography. J Am Coll Cardiol 1986;8:1341-7.
27. Lindsay Jr. J. Beall AC Jr, DeBakey ME, Diagnosis and treatment of disease of the aorta. In: Schlant R, Alexander RW, eds. Hurst's the heart, 9th edn. New York: McGraw-Hill, 1998:2461-82.
28. Lorenz CH, Walker ES, Morgan VL, et al. Normal human right and left ventricular mass, systolic function, and gender differences by cine magnetic resonance imaging. J Cardiovasc Magn Reson 1999;1:7-21.
29. Lund O. Preoperative risk evaluation and stratification of long-term survival after valve replacement for aortic stenosis. Reasons for earlier operative intervention. Circulation 1990;82:124-39.
30. Michel PL, ling B, Abou JS, et al. The effect of left ventricular systolic function on long-term survival in mitral and aortic regurgitation. J Heart Valve Dis 1995;4:Suppl 2:160-8.
31. Multicenter experience with balloon mitral commissurotomy. NHLBI Balloon Valvuloplasty Registry Participants. Circulation 1992;85:448-61.
32. Nadas AS, Ellison RC, Weidman WH. Report from the joint study on the Natural History of Congenital Heart Defect. Circulation 1977;56:11-187.
33. Nagel E, Lehmkuhl HB, Bocksch W, et al. Noninvasive diagnosis of ischemia-induced wall motion abnormalities with the use of high-dose dobutamine stress MRI: comparison with dobutamine stress echocardiography. Circulation 1999;99:763-70.
34. Nitenberg A, Foult JM, Antony I, et al. Coronary flow and resistance reserve in patients with chronic aortic regurgitation, angina pectoris and normal coronary arteries. J Am Coll Cardiol 1988;11:478-86.
35. O'Fallon WM, Weidman WJ. Long-term follow-up of congenital aortic stenosis, pulmonary stenosis, and ventricular septal defect: report from the Second Joint Study on the Natural History of Congenital Heart Defects (NHS-2). Circulation 1993;87:1-126.
36. Pruessmann KP, Weiger M, Scheidegger MB, et al. SENSE: Sensitivity encoding for fast MRI. Magn Reson Med 1999;42:952-62.
37. Rapaport E. Natural history of aortic and mitral valve disease. Am J Cardiol 1975;35:221-7.
38. Reimold SC, Maier SE, Fleischmann KE, et al. Dynamic nature of the aortic regurgitant orifice area during diastole in patients with chronic aortic regurgitation. Circulation 1994;89:2085-92.
39. Ross JJ. Afterload mismatch in aortic and mitral valve disease: implications for surgical therapy. J Am Coll Cardiol 1985;5:811-26.

40. Rowe JC, Bland EF, Sprague HB. The course of mitral stenosis without surgery: ten and twenty year perspectives. Ann Intern Med 1960;52:741-49.

41. Sakuma H, Globits S, Bourne MW, et al. Improved reproducibility in measuring LV volumes and mass using multicoil breath-hold cine MR imaging. J Magn Reson Imaging 1996;6:124-7.

42. Schwitter J. MR in valvular heart disease. Herz 2000; 25: 342-355.

43. Schwitter J, DeMarco T, Globits S, et al. Influence of felodipine on left ventricular hypertrophy and systolic function in orthotopic heart transplantant recipients: possible interaction with cyclosporine medication. J Heart Lung Transplant 1999;18:1003-13.

44. Schwitter J, Eberli FR, Ritter M, et al. Myocardial oxygen consumption in aortic valve disease with and without left ventricular dysfunction. Br Heart J 1992;67:161-9.

45. Scognamiglio R, Fasoli G, Dalla VS. Progression of myocardial dysfunction in aymptomatic patients with severe aortic insufficiency. Clin Cardiol 1986;9:151-6.

46. Scognamiglio R, Rahimtoola SH, Fasoli G, et al. Nifedipine in aymptomatic patients with severe aortic regurgitation and normal left ventricular function. N Engl J Med 1994;331:689-94.

47. Sechtem U, Pflugfelder PW, Cassidy MM, et al. Mitral or aortic regurgitation: quantification of regurgitant volumes with cine MR imaging. Radiology 1988;167:425-30.

48. Sheehan FH, Mitten LS, Factors influencing accuracy in left ventricular volume determintation. Am J Cardiol 1989;64:661-4.

49. Schellock FG. MR imaging of metallic implants and materials: a compilation of the literature. Am J Roentgenol 1988;151:811-4.

50. Siemienczuk D, Greenberg B, Morris C, et al. Chronic aortic insufficiency: factors associated with progression to aortic valve replacement. Ann Intern Med 1989;110:587-92.

51. Sondergaard L, Hildebrandt P, Lindvig K, et al. valve area and cardiac output in aortic stenosis: quantification by magnetic resonance velocity mapping. Am Heart J 1993;126:11576-64.

52. Sondergaard L, Lindvig K, Hildebrand P, et al. Quantification of aortic regurgitation by magnetic resonance velocity mapping. Am Heart J 1993;125:1081-90.

53. Soulen RL, Budinger TF, Higgins CB. Magnetic resonance imaging of prosthetic heart valves. Radiology 1985;154:705-7.

54. Spann JF, Bove AA, Natarajan G, et al. Ventricular performance, pump function and compensatory mechanisms in patients with aortic stenosis. Circulation 1980;62:576-82.

55. Summers RM, Andraskao BJ, Feuerstein IM, et al. Evaluation of the aortic root by MRI: insights from patients with homozygous familial hypercholesterolemia. Circulation 1998;98:509-18.

56. Teague SM, Heinsimer JA, Anderson JL, et al. Quantification of aortic regurgitation utilizing continuous wave Doppler ultrasound. J Am Coll Cardiol 1986;8:592-9.

57. The clinical role of magnetic resonance in cardiovascular disease. Task Force of the European Society of Cardiology, in collaboration with the Association of European Paediatric Cardiologists. Eur Heart J 1998;19:19-39.

58. Tribouilloy CM, Enriquez SM, Schaff HV, et al. Impact of preoperative symptoms on survival after surgical correction of organic mitral regurgitation: rationale for optimizing surgical indications. Circulation 1999:99:400-5.

59. Turina J, Hess O, Sepulcri F, et al. Spontaneous course of aortic valve disease. Eur Heart J 1987;8:471-83.

60. Walker PG, Oyre S, Pederson Em, et al. A new control volume method for calculating valvular regurgitation. Circulation 1995;92:579-86.

61. Xie GY, Berk MR, Smith MD, et al. A simplified method for determining regurgitant fraction by Doppler echocardiography in patients with aortic regurgitation. J Am Coll Cardiol 1994;24:1041-5.

62. Yang PC, Kerr AB, Liu AX, et al. New real-time interactive cardiac magnetic resonance imaging system complements echocardiography. J Am Coll Cardiol 1998;32:2049-56.

Section IV / Chapter 1

THE PLACE OF TISSUE VALVES IN AORTIC VALVE SURGERY

Prof.Dr. H.A. HUYSMANS

INTRODUCTION

A tissue valve has a more normal, undisturbed central flow pattern and no need for anticoagulation. therefore the interest for the use of tissue valves in aortic valve surgery dates back to the early days of valve surgery. in the early sixties the aortic homograft was introduced by ross and only shortly afterwards a porcine aortic xenograft was clinically used for the first time by binet[1]. in the late sixties ross performed the first autograft operation, in which the patients own pulmonary valve was implanted in the aortic position and a homograft was placed in the pulmonary position[2]. for several reasons the use of these valves remained restricted. homografts were not always easily procured and the first clinical results were disappointing in some less experienced centres, because of the technical difficulty of this procedure[1,3] Later it became apparent that good results with homografts were dependent on the right implantation technique. although it was thought that homografts were not very sensitive to rejection, it has meanwhile become clear that this can be a problem. nevertheless there has been a constant use of homografts and they have been of great value in paediatric cardiac surgery and in acute bacterial endocarditis.

PORCINE XENOGRAFTS

Porcine aortic xenografts were used either with a stent, to facilitate implantation, or stentless. In the beginning they failed early due to desintegration of the porcine tissue. After the introduction by Carpentier of glutaraldehyde fixation of the valve tissue the xenografts proved to be more durable. The stented xenografts became more popular and reached a peak in their use (up to 90 % of all valve prostheses in some centres) around the late seventies. Nevertheless the xenografts kept failing after some time and the need for re-operation with the connected risk made surgeons come back from its use (at present around 30 % of all cases) and return to mechanical valve prostheses. Studies on the causes of failure of tissue xenografts showed, that the treatment of tissues with glutaraldehyde and the changes in geometry were the main reasons for tissue calcification and degeneration, causing thickening of the leaflets, shrinking and tears and thereby regurgitation and stenosis.

Emboli may also occur, based on the degenerative lesions; these emboli seemed to be as frequent in patients with tissue valves not treated with anticoagulants as in patients with mechanical valves treated with anticoagulants. These processes occur earlier in younger patients. The durability in children and young adults may be as little as a few years only, but in patients over 70 years of age in the aortic position they can last 15 to 20 years. Biomechanical research has shown, that especially the use of a stent in tissue valves leads to very abnormal loading and bending stresses of the valve leaflets and that this stent might be the most important factor in tissue failure. The use of bovine pericardial tissue instead of porcine aorta did not really improve the results of tissue valves[4].

AUTOGRAFTS

The use of autografts remained restricted to a few centers. The technique seemed difficult and the concept of turning a one-valve disease into a two-valve lesion seemed strange. It was uncertain whether the pulmonary valve designed for a low pressure environment would be resistant enough to the high aortic pressure. The valve could distend and become regurgitant; there are however ways to avoid this. Only during the last decade surgeons became aware of the great value of autografts. They are primarily available in all patients, they have (normal?) growth potential in young children and can be used in almost all circumstances. The operative procedure however remains more complicated and time consuming and the disadvantages of a (pulmonary) homograft in the pulmonary artery remain.

EXPERIENCE AND USE OF TISSUE VALVES

Based on the experience of the first 15 years of use the indications for the use of tissue valves in aortic valve surgery during the past two decades were defined as follows: patients over 65 years of age, contra-indications for the use of anticoagulants, wish for pregnancy in young women (coumarin is teratogenic), bacterial endocarditis (?) and the specific wish of the patient. The results showed, that survival of patients with stented tissue valves was similar to those with mechanical valves, including the risk connected with re-operation. The use of autografts and homografts (= allografts) has been reserved for children and young adults and for cases of acute bacterial endocarditis.

Efforts have been made continuously to improve the quality of tissue valves and to make them more durable: new fixation methods (e.g. photofixation), anticalcification treatments (e.g. A.O.A.) and improved stent designs. So far the results of these changes have not been spectacular.

Around the mid-eighties when a better understanding of the failure mode of stented tissue valves became available and the good long-term results of homografts became known a renewed interest in homografts and stentless tissue valves developed. Experimental and clinical studies showed that these valves allowed an almost completely normal valve function with normal load and stresses of the leaflets, provided that the valve geometry was kept completely intact. This normal valve function allowed the heart muscle to return also to a completely normal function and LV mass. This is different from mechanical valves and stented tissue valves where some gradient remains and the left ventricle can never return to a completely normal function. The pressure curves always show a left ventricular pressure higher than the aortic pressure during end-systole, opposed to the normal pattern where it drops below aortic pressure at that time. Clinically this seems to lead to fewer valve related complications and better survival. So far there are only case-matched studies available. Randomized studies are on the way. It seems, that preserving the original geometry of the implanted valve, whether it is an autograft, a homograft or porcine aortic xenograft, is of vital importance to proper performance and durability. The choice of implantation technique is therefore essential. Subcoronary technique, whereby only the valve leaflets and commissure posts are implanted in the patients aorta (which usually has a different shape than the original valve aorta) makes it difficult to reconstruct the original geometry; it leads to a higher incidence of postoperative regurgitation. Total aortic root replacement allows maintenance of the original geometry best, but it is a bigger operation that needs re-implantation of the coronary arteries; it could have a higher complication rate and later re-operation might be difficult due to calcification of the aortic wall part of the graft. Root inclusion, implanting the complete graft in the patients aorta, leaves the geometry almost intact and does not need coronary re-implantation; the patients aortic wall protects the graft in case of re-operation. This technique however is the most difficult one of the three.

The obvious advantages of stentless valves make it necessary to reconsider the use of tissue valves in aortic valve surgery. One should ask the question whether a complete recovery of the heart, fewer valve related complications and a better survival allowing a completely normal life justify the use of a stentless (porcine) tissue valve rather than a mechanical valve prosthesis in younger patients, provided that no other heart disease is present. The total risk of a stentless valve, including the risk of re-operation(s) might be lower than that of a mechanical valve with anticoagulation. Theoretically the durability of a stentless valve should be considerably longer than that of any stented valve. We don't know however how long porcine tissue can survive intact after fixation; stented valves have already survived more than twenty years under favorable conditions. Another question that needs to be answered is when the stiffening and degeneration of a tissue valve starts;
re-operation is only performed when degeneration has caused serious deterioration of valve function, but long before that time the valve leaflets must have had stiffening that causes a less than optimal function. More sophisticated echo-Doppler studies might be able to answer this question.

INDICATIONS FOR THE USE OF TISSUE VALVES

The indications for tissue valves in aortic valve replacement at present should be as follows:

- In patients over 65 years of age a stentless porcine valve can be used; only when a fast, low risk procedure is needed the use of a stented tissue valve is justified.
- In infants and children the preference should be for a pulmonary autograft with pulmonary homograft replacement of the pulmonary valve or a homograft. If these are not available a mechanical valve would still be the best option.
- In bacterial endocarditis an autograft or homograft is the first choice. If these are not available a stentless porcine xenograft would be a good option.
- The indications in case of contra-indication for anticoagulation and in case a patient wants a tissue valve remain.

Changes in policy for patients under 65 years of age, now still considered for a mechanical valve should only be made with great care and in the context of a carefully conducted clinical trial.

REFERENCES

1. Binet JP, Duran CG, Carpentier A, Langlois J. Heterologous aortic valve transplantation. Lancet 1965; 2: 1275.
2. Ross DN Raplacement of aortic and mitral valves with a pulmonary autograft. Lancet 1967; 2: 956.
3. O' Brien MF, Clareborough JK Heterograft aortic valve transplantation for human valve disease Med. J. Aust. 1966; 2: 228-230.
4. Thrubikar M.J., Deck D., Aouad A., et al.: Role of mechanical stress in calcification of aortic bioprosthesis valves. J Thorac Cardiovasc Surg 86: 115-125, 1983.
5. Rousseau E.P.M.: Mechanical specifications for a closed leaflet valve prosthesis. Thesis Technical University Eindhoven, Wibro, Helmond, 1985
6. Christie G.W.: The anatomy of aortic heart valve leaflets: The influence of glutaraldehyde fixation on function. Eur J Cardiothorac Surg 6: S25-S33, 1992 (Suppl. 1)
7. Gott J.P., Pan Chih, Dorsey L.M.A., et al.: Calcification of porcine valves: A successful new method of antimineralisation. Ann Thorac Surg 53: 207-216, 1992
8. Moore M.A., Mc Illroy B.K., Philips R.E. jr.: Nonaldehyde sterilization of biological tissue for use in implantable medical devices. ASAIOJ 43: 23-30, 1997
9. Jamieson W.R.E., Burr L.H., Miyagishima R.T., et al.: Actuarial versus actual freedom from structural valve deterioration with the Carpentier-Edwards porcine bioprosthesis. Can J Cardiol 15 (9): 973-978, 1999
10. Langley S.M., McGuirk S.P., Chaudry M.A., et al.: Twenty year follow-up of aortic valve replacement with antibiotic sterilized homografts in 200 patients. Seminars Thorac Cardiovasc Surg 11: 28-34, 1999 (Suppl. 1)
11. Hazekamp M.G., Goffin Y.A., Huysmans H.A.: The value of the stentless biovalve prosthesis: An experimental study. Eur J Cardiothorac Surg 7: 514-519, 1993
12. Del Rizzo D., Abdoh A., Cartier P., et al.: The effect of prosthetic valve type on s survival after aortic valve surgery. Seminars Thorac Cardiovasc Surg 11: 1-8, 1999 (Suppl. 1)
13. Walter T., Falk V., Langebartels G., et al.: Regression of left ventricular hypertrophy after stentless versus conventional aortic valve replacement. Seminars Thorac Cardiovasc Surg 11: 18-21, 1999 (Suppl. 1)
14. Oury J.H., Mackey S.K., Duran C.M.: Critical analysis of the Ross procedure: Do its problems justify wider application? Seminars Thorac Cardiovasc Surg 11:55-61, 1999 (Suppl. 1)
15. Jin X.Y., Westaby S., Gibson D.G., et al.: Left ventricular remodeling and improvement in "Freestyle" stentless valve haemodynamics. Eur J Cardiothorac Surg 12: 63-69, 1997
16. Kon N.D., Cordell A.R., Adair S.M., et al.: Comparison of results using "Freestyle" stentless porcine bioprosthesis with cryopreserved aortic root allograft. Seminars Thorac Cardiovasc Surg 11: 69-73, 1999 (Suppl. 1)
17. Barratt-Boyes B.G., Christie G.W., Raudkivi P.J.: The stentless bioprosthesis: Surgical challenges and implications for long-term durability. Eur J Cardiothor Surg 6: S156-159, 1992 (Suppl. 1)
18. Westaby S., Huysmans H.A., David T.E.: Stentless aortic bioprosthesis: Compelling data from the Second International Symposium. Ann Thorac Surg 65: 235-240, 1998

THE PLACE OF THE ROSS PROCEDURE IN AORTIC VALVE DISEASE

Prof.Dr. M. HAZEKAMP, P. SCHOOF

INTRODUCTION

Donald Ross was the first to clinically apply the concept of replacing the aortic valve with the pulmonary autograft in 1967.[1] His goal was to have a permanent and durable substitute for the diseased aortic valve in young adults with isolated aortic valve disease. In his own words " a permanent valve would avoid the dangers of a long-term anticoagulation with mechanical valves and increasingly hazardous repeat bioprosthetic valve operations at 10- to 15-year intervals"[2].

For many years Mr. Ross has remained a lonely pioneer. Other surgeons have waited a long time to follow his example. Only in the last 10 years the Ross procedure has expanded rapidly: an increasing number of surgeons learned to use the technique and the indications for its use were extended.
The maximal follow-up of the Ross operation is now 33 years. When we look back we will see that the original method of subcoronary implantation has been replaced for the technique of "full root replacement" with a very recent tendency to return to the original way of placing the pulmonary autograft inside the patients' own aortic root.[3] We will observe that the Ross operation is now used in all age groups ranging from newborns to elderly patients.[4,5] In the pediatric age group other indications than isolated aortic valve disease may form a reason for the Ross procedure, e.g. tunnel-form obstruction of the left ventricular outflow tract.[6] Even patients with destructive bacterial endocarditis of the aortic valve and the surrounding tissues have been successfully treated by this operation.[7]

The Ross procedure has many advantages but also certain disadvantages. With time we will learn with more precision to define the best indications for this daring concept.

112

TECHNICAL ASPECTS

Fundamentally, the Ross procedure consists in replacing the aortic valve by the patients' pulmonary valve. The original operations performed by mr. Ross were subcoronary or so-called freehand implantations of the pulmonary autograft: the pulmonary valve was scalloped and placed inside the aortic root of the patient.

Elkins was one of the first surgeons to use the technique of root replacement. The whole aortic root together with the diseased aortic valve is removed and replaced by the adjacent pulmonary trunk.[8] The coronary arteries are reimplanted in the corresponding sinuses of the autograft. The wall of the new aortic root will then be a pulmonary artery wall.

The technique of root replacement is easier to reproduce and the risk of postoperative aortic incompetence is less than if the technique of subcoronary implantation is used. Size differences between aortic and pulmonary valves can be solved better with root replacement. If the aortic valve annulus is smaller than the pulmonary valve diameter, it may be widened by incising into the muscular septum or aorto-mitral fibrous continuity. If the aortic annulus is too wide to fit the pulmonary valve, its diameter is reduced by a pursestring suture or by commissural plication sutures.

A third technique besides the techniques of subcoronary aortic valve replacement and aortic root replacement is the root inclusion method where the pulmonary trunk geometry is better preserved than with the subcoronary technique. With the root inclusion technique the pulmonary trunk is placed as a cylinder inside the patients' own aortic root.

If the subaortic region is narrow an extended Ross operation may be necessary: the septum is incised and the left ventricular outflow tract is augmented by placing a patch in the incised septum. At the same time excessive fibrous and/ or muscular tissue may be resected.

Care should be taken to avoid damage to the first septal artery when releasing the pulmonary trunk from the right ventricle.[9] By using a proper technique and with sufficient experience it is not necessary to localize this artery by angiography preoperatively.

The defect in the right ventricular outflow tract is repaired by a slightly oversized cryopreserved pulmonary homograft. Alternative conduits are aortic homografts or stentless porcine valved conduits.

ADVANTAGES

No anticoagulants are needed, no thrombo-embolism is encountered and the chance of autograft or homograft endocarditis is very low. A gradient free reconstruction is possible in almost all types of pathology. Rejection or calcific degeneration of the autograft does not occur. The pulmonary autograft has proven to withstand the systemic pressure. In children the pulmonary autograft is the only aortic valve substitute that grows with the child. The reoperation rate for the right-sided homografts is low, lower than that of extracardiac conduits that are used to repair different forms of congenital heart disease.[10] Current operative mortality is as low as for implantation of other aortic valve prostheses.

DISADVANTAGES

The Ross procedure is a long procedure with an average aortic cross-clamp time of 2 hours. Therefore, if other procedures are to be performed simultaneously with aortic valve replacement, the Ross procedure is not always the best choice as myocardial ischemia time may become too long. Thus patients who also need coronary artery bypass grafting are usually not optimal candidates for the Ross procedure. Furthermore, most connective tissue disorders such as Marfan's syndrome and systemic lupus erythematodes form a contraindication for the Ross operation as the pulmonary valve may also be affected by these disorders. In rheumatic valve disease the pulmonary autograft has been reported to become involved in the inflammation process following the Ross procedure.[11] Furthermore, following the Ross procedure two valvular replacements are at risk instead of only one. The long-term fate of the pulmonary autograft is not completely known as the number of long-term survivors is still limited.

RESULTS

In the International Ross Registry as maintained by dr.J.Oury a total of 4071 patients are included.[12] Thirty percent of the patients was operated at a age less than 20 years. The mean age at operation was 30,7 years ranging from 0 to 79 years. The subcoronary implant technique was used in 13,7 %, the root inclusion method in 6,7 % and the root replacement technique in the remaining majority of the patients. In 66 % of the patients follow-up was complete with a maximum follow-up of 25 years.

The operative mortality (< 30 days) was 4,0 %. Ross operations in small babies are included in this series. This may indicate that the mortality in young adults is less, as has been published by others.[3, 5,13,14] In a well-documented group of 2610 patients with a follow-up of maximal 25 years, freedom from pulmonary autograft explantation is 90 % at 10 years and 82 % at 25 years (with 207 patients remaining at risk after 10 years and 33 patients after 25 years). In this same group freedom from right ventricular outflow tract repair or replacement was 91 % at 10 years and 84 % after 25 years.

The incidence of autograft reoperation is dependent of several technical factors. If the subcoronary technique is used to implant the pulmonary autograft the experience of the surgeon is of importance as this technique is more subject to surgical technical errors. Although not proven yet, the method of root inclusion is probably less likely to suffer from technical failure as here the pulmonary autograft geometry is better preserved. The root replacement technique is more reproducible and the chance of autograft incompetence is less than that if the other two techniques have been used.[15]

Some reports mention a small incidence of aneurysmatic dilatation of the pulmonary autograft root.[3,15] This phenomenon occurs solely following the technique of root replacement as the pulmonary wall is more elastic than the aortic wall.[16] This dilatation may be prevented by performing the proximal anastomosis between the autograft root and aortic annulus with a supporting strip of autologous pericardium or Teflon. Dilatation at the level of the sinotubular junction can be avoided in the same way by adding a strip of pericardium or Teflon in the distal suture line.

COMMENT

With careful patient selection the Ross procedure is a good way of treatment of aortic valve disease. Long-term results are excellent with low reoperation rates for the pulmonary autograft and the right-sided homograft conduit.

Reoperation to replace a right-sided conduit is easy and possible with a very low morbidity and mortality. An incompetent pulmonary autograft may be repaired with lasting results in an important percentage.

The pulmonary valve is a hemodynamically perfect substitute for the aortic valve with natural valve behavior, absolute absence of gradients and a very low incidence of serious valve incompetence. Thrombo-embolism is almost zero following the Ross operation and the likelihood of postoperative endocarditis is very low. Furthermore, the pulmonary autograft is the only growing valve substitute available for the pediatric age group. The Ross operation is the best solution for combined aortic valve pathology in neonates and young infants. Difficult problems such as tunnel obstructions of the left ventricular outflow tract may now be treated by extended pulmonary autograft root replacement with septal patch augmentation.

Nevertheless, a word of caution should be added as a good outcome of the Ross procedure depends on several factors. The technique is more difficult than aortic valve replacement by mechanical or biological valve prosthesis and a certain learning curve is thus present. Implantation by subcoronary or root inclusion techniques prevents later aortic root dilatation but these techniques are somehow more likely to produce postoperative valve incompetence. The method of root replacement is easier to reproduce with almost no valve insufficiency but some reports mention a small percentage of later root dilatation.[3,15,17] More and longer follow-up studies will be necessary to define the best technical way to perform the Ross procedure in adults.

REFERENCES

1. Ross DN. Replacement of aortic and mitral valves with a pulmonary autograft. Lancet 2: 956 (1967)
2. Ross D, Jackson M, Davies J. Pulmonary autograft aortic valve replacement: long-term results. J Cardiac Surg 6: 529-33 (1991)
3. David TE, Omran A, Ivanov J, Armstrong S, de Sa MPL, Sonnenberg B, Webb G. Dilation of the pulmonary autograft after the Ross procedure. J Thorac Cardiovasc Surg 119: 210-20 (2000)
4. Elkins RC, Knott-Craig CJ, Ward KE, Lane MM. The Ross operation in children: 10-year experience. Ann Thorac Surg 65: 496-502 (1998)
5. Stelzer P, Weinrauch S, Tranbaugh RF. Ten years experience with the modified Ross procedure. J Thorac Cardiovasc Surg 115: 1091-100 (1998)
6. Daenen W, Gewillig M. Extended aortic root replacement with pulmonary autografts. Eur J Cardiothorac Surg 7: 42-6 (1993)
7. Petterson G, Tingleff J, Joyce FS. Treatment of aortic valve endocarditis with the Ross operation. Eur J Cardiothorac Surg 13: 678-84 (1998)
8. Elkins RC, Santangelo K, Stelzer P, Randolph JD, Knott-Craig CJ. Pulmonary autograft replacement of the aortic valve: an evolution of technique. J Cardiac Surg 7: 108-16 (1992)
9. Melo JQ, Abecassis ME, Neves JS, et al. Can the location of the large septal artery be predicted? Eur J Cardiothorac Surg 9: 628-30 (1995)
10. Willems TP, Bogers AJ, Cromme-Dijkhuis AH, Steyenberg EW, van Herwerden L, Hokken RB, Hess J, Bos E. Allograft reconstruction of the right ventricular outflow tract. Eur J Cardiothorac Surg 10:609-14 (1996)
11. Al-Halees Z, Kumar N, Gallo R, Gometza B, Duran CMG. Pulmonary autograft for aortic valve replacement in rheumatic disease: a caveat. Ann Thorac Surg 60: Suppl: 172-6 (1995)
12. Oury JH, Hiro SP, Maxwell JM, Lamberti JJ, Duran CG. The Ross procedure: current registry results. Ann Thorac Surg 66 (Suppl): 162-5 (1998)
13. Rubay JE, Buche M, El Khoury GA, Vanoverschelde J-LJ, Sluysmans T, Marchandise B, J-C Schoevaerdts, RA Dion. The Ross operation: Mid-term results. Ann Thorac Surg 67: 1355-8 (1999)
14. Braun J, Hazekamp MG, Schoof PH, Ottenkamp J, Huysmans HA. Short-term follow-up of the Ross operation in children. J Heart Valve Dis 7: 615-9 (1998)
15. Elkins RC, Lane MM, McCue C. Pulmonary autograft reoperation: incidence and management. Ann Thorac Surg 62: 450-5 (1996)
16. Schoof PH, Hazekamp MG, van Wermeskerken GK, de Heer E, Bruijn JA, Gittenberger-de Groot AC, Huysmans HA. Disproportionate enlargement of the pulmonary autograft in the aortic position. J Thorac Cardiovasc Surg 115: 1264-72 (1999).
17. Schmidtke C, Bechtel JFM, Hueppe M, Noetzold A, Sievers H-H. Size and distensibility of the aortic root and aortic valve function after different techniques of the Ross procedure. J Thorac Cardiovasc Surg 119: 990-7 (2000).

IS A MECHANICAL PROSTHESIS ALWAYS THE BEST SOLUTION FOR AN AORTIC VALVE REPLACEMENT IN ADULTS?

A.H.M. VAN STRATEN

INTRODUCTION

In order for a valve prosthesis to be perfect, the prosthesis should have a hemodynamic performance similar to a healthy native aortic valve, no valve related long-term morbidity and mortality, should be easy to implant, should last forever and should have a good availability in all sizes. None of the valve prostheses, that are available today, fulfill all of these criteria. When a patient needs an aortic valve replacement today, there are several options for the valve substitute. The most often used options are: mechanical prosthesis (MP) "bileaflet" or "tilting disk", porcine or pericardial bioprosthesis (BP), porcine or pericardial stentless bioprosthesis (SBP), homograft (allograft) (HG) and pulmonary autograft (PA). In order to determine which of these is the best valve prosthesis for a particular patient, we cannot rely on large prospective randomized studies proving that at any given age of a patient one kind of valve prosthesis is superior to all others. The reason for this is that such studies are not available. Therefore, we have to look at the results of different kind of valve substitutes in large mainly retrospective series. It is important to realize that it is very difficult to compare the reported results. Reports of long-term results of aortic valve replacement with different kind of valve prostheses may differ in methodology and statistics. Moreover, most reports are coming from different countries, are done by different investigators whereas patient populations are often not comparable. Only the use of different statistical methods may lead to important differences in outcome[1]. The different aspects of a valve substitute, determining which is the best are: hemodynamic performance, long-term valve related morbidity, long-term valve related death, availability, easiness to implant the prosthesis and comfort for the patient.

HEMODYNAMIC PERFORMANCE

One study showed that HG, as compared with MP, provided significantly better hemodynamic performance, leading to better regression of the LV hypertrophy [2].
Another study showed that hemodynamic performance of HG as well as of SBP results in more extensive reduction of left ventricular hypertrophy and greater improvement of left ventricular function than with MP or BP [3]. Another study suggested that after HG implantation patients more often continued professional activity than after MP implantation [4]. The pressure gradient over a SBP is very low and improving over time [5].

VALVE RELATED MORBIDITY

Thrombo-embolism (TE), valve thrombosis (VT) and bleeding (BL)
An INR between 2 and 4.9 leads to the lowest incidence of TE plus BL[6]. In a well organized country as the Netherlands, where the target INR in aortic valve replacement patients should be between 2,5 and 4, only 50 % of all INR's in a group of 200 of our MP patients appeared to be in this range during follow-up (not published). In some studies older age was shown to be a risk factor for TE as well as for BL [6,7]. In another study, age was not a risk factor [8].

Mechanical valves
No studies with large numbers of patients and long-term follow-up are available, indicating that a particular mechanical valve prosthesis is superior to the world-wide most implanted MP. Therefore we look at the results of the "st Jude" mechanical prosthesis for the rate of TE and BL in patients with an MP. The linearized risk of all TE is 2.3 - 2.5% per patient-year [9,10,11]. TE may lead to several situations: death, permanent impairment or full recovery. Freedom from permanent valve related impairment after 15 years in one study was 83 %[11]. In another study it was 79 % after 10 years [9]. The linearized rate for valve thrombosis was 0.1-0.3 %. The linearized rates for bleeding in the same studies were 2.0 – 2,2 % per patient-year.

Bioprostheses
For BP we analyzed studies about the Carpentier-Edwards porcine bioprosthesis, the Carpentier-Edwards pericardial bioprosthesis and the Hancock II bioprosthesis. Linearized rate for TE is 1.7 - 2.4 and for BL 0.3-0.6 [12,13,14,15]. VT is not mentioned in the previously mentioned studies. Long-term follow-up of one of the stentless valves (Toronto SPV) after 8 years showed, that the risk for TE with SBP was statistically not different from the risk with the Hancock II bioprosthesis, but the follow-up is only 8 years and the number of patients is relatively small [16].

Stentless, bioprostheses, homografts and autografts
Risk for TE with HG and AG is low [17,18,19]. In a group of 275 HG patients, with a mean follow-up of 4.5 years, were only 3 episodes of thrombo-embolism [19]. The risk for TE plus BL is higher with MP than with BP and SBP. The risk is probably lowest with HG and AG though till now there is no absolute proof for that.

Periprosthetic leak (Non structural dysfunction)
Linearized risk for periprosthetic leak with MP is 0.2-0.3 [10,20]. With BP 0.4-0.5 [12,14]. With proper technique periprosthetic leak in SBP, HG and AG should be very low or even absent in case of total root replacement.
Risk for periprosthetic leak appeared to be the same after MP and BP implantation and lower after SBP, HG and AG implantation.

Prosthetic valve endocarditis
The reported risk for prosthetic endocarditis with MP is 0.2 –0.4 [9,10,11,20]. With BP the reported risk is 0.5-0.8 [12,13,14,15]. The reported risk with HG is 0.5 [18,19]. Freedom from prosthetic endocarditis with SBP after 8 years is 98%[16]. The freedom from prosthetic valve endocarditis at 15 years with HG was 94% [21,22]. The risk in MP and BP appeared to have an early peak[22]. Compared to HG and to MP the risk in BP patients in one study was higher [22].

Structural valve failure
Structural failure for modern MP is not reported. In BP durability was better when the valve was implanted in the aortic position and for patients with older age [12,13,14,15]. Freedom from structural valve deterioration after 18 years in patients older than 70 years with a Carpentier-Edwards bioprosthesis was 82 %, whereas for a patient with the same valve aged between 41 and 50 years it was 25 %[12]. In HG freedom from degenerative valve failure at 10 years was 89% in a patient group with a mean age of 45 years[19]. Crypreserved homografts showed better durability than homografts stored at 4 degrees C [21]. Actuarial freedom from valve deterioration after 15 years with cryopreserved homografts was 80% in a group of patients with a mean age of 54 years (3-80 years) [22]. Durability of SBP and AG has yet to be established. In general it is noted that MP are durable and BP SBP and HG and probably AG not.

Hemolysis
Despite the fact that hemolysis is a rare clinical problem after aortic valve replacement with any kind of prosthesis, postoperative LDH level is significantly more elevated in patients after MP implantation than after BP, HG, AG, or SBP implantation.

Freedom from reoperation
After MP implantation the linearized risk for reoperation is 0.4-1% per patient-year leading to freedom from reoperation after 15 years of 91 % [9,10,11,20]. Risk for reoperation in BP is 2,7% per patient-year leading to freedom from reoperation in BP after 10 years of 91% and after 15 years of 51-71% [12,13,14,15]. In HG patients the freedom from re-operation after 10 years was 91%[19] and 69% after 15 years in another study[22]. Reasons for reoperation in HG as a percentage of all reoperations are: structural valve deterioration 35%, endocarditis 21% and technical failure 44% [22]. In SBP patients the freedom from reoperation at 8 years was 98% [16]. Since structural valve deterioration is likely to increase after 8 years, this number will probably increase. Because of the more demanding surgical technique, the risk of early reoperation depends on the experience of the surgeon. In our series of 175 stentless aortic valves, with a maximum follow-up of 6 years, we had 4 early reoperations. Two, because of improper sizing or improper technique and two, because of problems with the coronary ostiae, 6 months postoperatively. In a reported group of 680 HG patients 22 had early aortic incompetence leading to 14 reoperations [22]. With proper technique and proper timing of the reoperatieon the risk of a reoperation for structural valve deterioration can be as low as 4.3-4.8 % [14,23].

VALVE RELATED DEATH

Age at the time of implant and concomitant diseases are important risk factors for late non-valve related death. We will look at valve-related death instead of over-all survival. Reported freedom from valve-related death in MP after 15 years is 78% in one series [11]. Causes of valve related death were as a percentage of all valve related deaths: sudden death 10-29%, valve thrombosis 4%, endocarditis 19-20%, cerebral embolism 10-14%, cerebral bleed 9-50%, cardiac tamponade 4%, others/unknown 17 % [10-11]. After 15 years a linearized risk for valve-related death in a BP group was 1-1.6 % per patient-year including the risk of a reoperation [12,14]. Causes of death in a combined aortic and mitral BP group as a percentage of total valve related deaths were: anticoagulant related bleeding 9-10%, non-structural dysfunction 5-6%, prosthetic endocarditis 11-18%, structural valve dysfunction 20-36 %, thrombo-embolism 23-46 %, sudden death 21% [12-14]. In a case-control study freedom from cardiac mortality after 8 years was significantly better after SBP implantation than after BP implantation: 95 versus 81% [24]. After HG and AG implantation the reported survival in a relatively young patient group was very good [17,19,25]. Most of these studies do not mention valve-related death separately.

AVAILABILITY

Availability is a problem only for HG and therefore also for PA. The pulmonary valve, which is used in the aortic position, is mostly replaced by HG.

IMPLANTATION TECHNIQUE

Technique for implanting an MP and a BP is similar and compared to techniques to implant SBP, HG or AG, relatively simple. There are several techniques for implanting a SBP or a HG [26]. The commonly used techniques are (modified) subcoronary implantation, root inclusion technique and full root replacement. All these techniques are more difficult and more time consuming than the technique for implanting a mechanical prosthesis or a stented bioprosthesis. The technique for implanting a pulmonary autograft is even more difficult [27]. This leads to longer operative time, with longer ischemic (cross-clamp) time but not leading to more operative death [17]. Technical failure can lead to valve incompetence and early reoperation [22].

COMFORT FOR THE PATIENT

Mechanical prostheses are making noise. In a group of 100 patients with a st Jude MP, that we investigated, 17 patients did complain about the noise (not published). Others reported also a negative impact of valve sounds on the quality of live of patients and his or her relatives [28]. Also the constant need to take medication and to control the level of anti-coagulation, being inevitable after implantation of MP, has a negative impact on quality of live.

DISCUSSION

There is no absolute proof of the superiority of one kind of valve substitute. Studies comparing the results after MP and BP implantation at older age are coming to opposite conclusions: to use more MP in older patients [29] or to use more BP in older patients [30]. A study comparing results after HG versus MP implantation in young patients suggested better results after MP implantation [31]. A lot of questions are still unanswered. Will MP last forever? Does the pattern of flow across a heart valve have an effect on coronary flow or ventricular function? Is a rigid ring in the aortic annulus detrimental for ventricular function? Does a residual pressure gradient have a late effect? Is the relatively large proportion of sudden death with MP and BP caused by the hemodynamic performance of the MP or BP? Will the better hemodynamic performance of the SBP, HG and AG lead to less sudden death and to better overall survival? Can the target INR safely be lowered as suggested in one study [32], knowing that less than 50 % of patients INR's are in that target range? Will new MP designs allow further lowering of the INR? Is it possible that the patient himself can regulate his INR as good as or even better than his doctor? Can every surgeon perform implantation of HG or SBP with the same operative results as for BP or MP implantation? When we implant BP or SBP or HG now and the patient comes for a reoperation in 12-15 years, will we have a superior substitute at that time? Will new anti-calcification treatment of BP lead to better durability?

Furthermore in making the choice for a valve substitute, we have to consider the age of the patient, concomitant operative procedures such as coronary artery bypass surgery, the lifestyle and other diseases of the patient. Do we have to weigh the risk of 25 or 30 years of TE and BL in MP against the reduced risk of TE and BL plus the risk of one reoperation in BP in a patient with a life expectancy of 30 years or more? If the risk of TE and BL is reduced in younger as compared with older patients, the MP, implanted in a younger patient, will be still in if that patient is older. Even if we had all the answers and could calculate the prognosis after implantation of each of the different valve substitutes, the patient might choose for an option other than the calculated best. Because consequences of a choice may interfere with the lifestyle of the patient, it is important to explain the advantages and disadvantages of the different kind of valve prostheses. The patient and not the surgeon will have to live with the consequences of a particular choice. A patient might prefer a reoperation in 12 or 15 years without anti-coagulant medication in the meantime. In those 12-15 years he can make a sailing trip around the world. Another patient might do anything to avoid a reoperation.

REFERENCES

1. Grunkemeier GL, Li H, Starr A. Heart valve replacement: a statistical review of 35 years' result. J Heart Valve Dis 1999:8:466-71
2. Basarir S, Islamoglu F, Ozkisacik E, Atay Y, Boga M, Bakalim T, Ozbaran M,Telli A. Comparative analysis of left ventricular hemodynamics and hy pertrophy after aortic valve replacement with homografts or mechanical valves. J Heart Valve Dis 2000;9:45-52
3. Jin XY, Zhang Z, Gibson DG, Yacoub MH, Pepper JR. Effects of valve substitute on change in left ventricular function and hypertrophy after aortic valve replacement. Ann Thorac Surg 1996;62:683-90
4. Podolec P, Wierzbicki K, Olszowska M, Woickiewicz T, Pfitzner R, Tracz W, Dziatkowiak. A Comparison of quality of life, physical and professional activity in patients after homogenous versus mechanic aortic valve replacement. Kardiol Pol 1997;47/10:310-16
5. Bauer LH, Jin XY, Houdas Y, Peels CH, Braun J, Kappetein AP, Prat A, Hazekamp MG, Van Straten BH, Ploeg A, Sieders A, Voogd PJ, Bruschke AV, van de Wall EE, Westaby S, Huysmans HA. Echocardiographic parameters of the freestyle stentless bioprosthesis in aortic position: the European experience. J Am Soc Echocardigr 1999;12:729-35
6. Cannegieter SC, Rosendaal FR, Wintzen AR, van der Meer FJM, Vandenbroucke JP, Briet E. Optimal oral anticoagulant therapy in patients with mechanical heart valves. N Eng J Med 1995;333:11-7
7. Jamieson WRE, Miyagishima RT, Grunkemeier GL, Germann E, Henderson C, Lichtenstein SV, Ling H, Munro AI. Bileafler mechanical prostheses for aortic valve replacement in patients younger than 65 years and 65 years of age or older: Major thromboembolic and hemorrhagic complications. Can . J. Surg 1999:42/1:27-36
8. Masters RG, Semelhago LC, Pipe AL, Keon WJ. Are older patients with mechanical heart valves at increased risk. Ann Thorac Surg 1999;68:2169-72
9. Kahn S, Chaux A, Matlof J, Blanche C, DeRobertis M, Kass R, Tsai TP, Tranto A, Nessim S, Gray R, Czer L. The st Jude valve. Experience with 1000 cases. J Thorac Cardiovasc Surg 1994;108:1010-20
10. Ibrahim M, O'Kane H, Cleland J, Gladstone D, Sarsam M, Patterson C. The st Jude valve prosthesis. A thirteen-year experience. J Thorac Cardiovasc Surg 1994;108:221-30
11. Zellner JL, Kratz JM, CrumbleyIII AJ, Stroud MR, Bradley SM, Sade RM, Crawford FA. Long-term experience with the st Jude Medical valve prosthesis. Ann Thorac Surg 1999;68:1210-8
12. Jamieson WR, Burr LH, Munro AI, Miyagishima RT. Carpentier-Edwards Standard porcine bioprosthesis: A 21-year experience. Ann Thorac Surg 1998;66:S40-3
13. Glower DD, Landolfo KP, Cherruvu S, Cen Y, Harrison JK, Bashore TM, Smith PK Jones RH,Wolfe WG, Lowe JE. Determinants of 15-year outcome with 1119 standard Carpentier-Edwards porcine valves. Ann Thorac Surg 1998;66:S44-8
14. Jamieson WR, Ling H, Burr LH, Fradet GJ, Miyagishima RT., Janusz MT, Lichtenstein SV. Carpentierr-Edwards supraannular porcine bioprosthesis evaluation over 15 years. Ann Thorac Surg 1998;66:S49-52
15. Poirer NC, Pelletier LC, Pellerrin M, Carrier M. 15-Year experience with the Carpentier-Edwards pericardial bioprosthesis. Ann Thorac Surg 1998;66:S57-61
16. David TE, Armstrong S, Sun Z. The Hancock II bioprosthesis at 12 years. Ann Thorac Surg 1998;66:S95-8
17. Aklog L. Carr-White GS, Birks EJ, Yacoub MH. Pulmonary autograft verrsus aortic homograft for aortic valve replacement: interim results from a prospective randomized trial. J Heart Valve Dis 2000;9:176-189

124

18. Kirklin JK, Smith D, Novick W, Naftel DC, Kirklin JW, Pacifico AD, Nanda NC,, Helmcke FR, Bourge RC. Long-term function of cryopreserved aortic homografts. A ten-year study. J Thorac Surg 1993;106:154-66

19. Yacoub M, Rasmi NRH, Sundt TM, Lund O, Boyland E, Radley-Smith R, Kharghani A, Mitchell A. Fourteen-year experience with homovital homografts for aortic valve replacement. J Thorac Cardiovasc Surg 1995;110:186-94

20. Czer LS Chaux A, Matlof JM, DeRobertis MA, Nessim SA, Scarlata D, Khan SS, Kass RM, Tsai TP, Blanche C, Gray RJ. Ten-Year experience with the st Jude Medical valve for primary valve replacement. J Thorac Cardiovasc Surg 1990;100:44-55

21. Agnihotri AK, McGiffin DC, Galbraith AJ, O'Brian MF. The prevalence of infective endocarditis after aortic valve replacement. J Thorac Cardiovasc Surg 1995;110:1708-24

22. O'Brien MF, Stafford EG, Gardner MA, Pohlner PG, Tesar PJ, Cochrane AD, Mau TK, Gall KL, Smith SE. Allograft aortic valve replacement: long-term follow-up. Ann Thorac Surg 1995 60(2supll):S65-70

23. Akins CW, Buckley MJ, Dagget WM, Hilgenberg AD, Vlahakes GJ, Torchiana DF, Madsen JC. Risk of reoperative valve replacement for failed mitral and aortic bioprostheses. Ann Thorac Surg 1998;65:1545-51

24. David TE, Puschmann R, Ivanov J, Bos J, Armstrong S, Feindel CM, Scully HE. Aortic valve replacement with stentless and stented porcine valves: a case matched study. J Thorac Cardiovasc Surg;1998;116:235-41

25. Moidl R, Simon P, Aschauer C, Chevtchik O, Kupilik N, Rodler S, Wolner E, Laufer G. Does the Ross operation fulfil the objective performance criteria established for new prosthetic heart valves? J Heart Valve Dis 2000;9:190-94

26. Barret-Boyes BG, Christie GW, Raudkivi PJ. The stentless bioprosthesis: surgical challanges and implications for long-term durability. Eur J Cardio-thorac Surg 1992;6:S39-43

27. Ross DN, Replacement of aortic and mitral valves with a pulmonary autograft. Lancet 1967;2:956-58

28. Blome-Eberwein S.A., Mrowinski D, Hofmeister J, Hetzer R. Impact of mechanical heart valves prosthesis sound on patients' quality of live. Ann. Thorac. Surg 1996;61/2:594-602

29. Milano A, Guglielmi C, De Carlo M, Di Gregorio O, Borzoni G, Verunelli F, Bortolli U. Valve-related complications in elderly patients with biological and mechanical aortic valves. Ann Thorac Surg 1998;66/6:S82-87

30. Davis EA, Green PS, Cameron, DE, Gott VL, Laschinger JC, Struart RS, Sussman MS, Watkins L,Baymgartner WA. Bioprosthetic versus mechanical prostheses for aortic replacement in the elderly. Circulation 1996;94/9:SII121-II125

31. Gross C. Klima U, Mair R, Brucke P. Aortic homografts versus mechanical valves in aortic valve replacement in young patients: A retrospective study. Ann Thorac Surg 1998;66/6:S194-197

32. Horstkotte D, Schulte HD, Bircks W, Strauer BE. Lower intensity anticoagulation therapy results in lower complication rate with the st Jude Medical prosthesis. J Cardiovasc Surg 1994;107:1136-45

POSTOPERATIVE REGRESSION OF LEFT VENTRICULAR HYPERTROPHY

Dr. L.H.B. BAUR, C.H. PEELS, J. KOOIKER, Prof.Dr. H.A. HUYSMANS

INTRODUCTION

Long lasting valvular disease has considerable impact on left ventricular chamber geometry and myocardial function. Changes in left ventricular function, volume and mass are dependent on the responsible valve, and the disease state (stenosis or insufficiency). If the valve defect is corrected, before the left ventricular myocardium has been irreversibly damaged, changes of myocardial structure and function will ultimately return to normal. However, if valvular disease is corrected too late, left ventricular dysfunction will persist. Changes of ventricular geometry and mass differ for the various disease entities and will therefore be discussed separately.

AORTIC STENOSIS

Aortic valve stenosis is associated with chronic pressure overload. In patients with aortic stenosis in the compensated stage, this process is accompanied by an adaptive increase of left ventricular mass with a preserved left ventricular enddiastolic volume and stroke volume[1,2]. Ventricular hypertrophy in aortic stenosis involves both the muscular and nonmuscular compartments of the left ventricle[3] and is assumed to result from parallel addition of new myofibrils[4] and an increase of interstitial tissue. The gain of left ventricular muscle and interstitial tissue will initially result in diastolic dysfunction[3]. Longstanding severe pressure or volume overload, however, will ultimately result in myocardial depression with reduced stroke volume but still no irreversible myocardial damage[20]. This process, also know as "afterload mismatch"[5] can readily be reversed by lowering afterload. If aortic valve disease is not corrected in this stage, irreversible myocardial damage may occur with persistent left ventricular dysfunction even if the aortic valve has been replaced. Characteristic differences in evolution of left ventricular function and left ventricular hypertrophy in patients with aortic stenosis have been reported between women and men. Women with aortic stenosis have a characteristic pattern of concentric left ventricular hypertrophy with a smaller, thicker-walled chamber compared with an eccentric pattern of hypertrophy and chamber dilation observed in men[6]. With similar degrees of left ventricular outflow obstruction, cardiac performance is frequently more depressed in men than it is in women[6].

Preoperative left ventricular function and the pattern of left ventricular hypertrophy have been shown to be the most important determinants of survival among patients undergoing aortic valve replacement[7,8]. Aortic valve surgery results in immediate reduction in preload and afterload[9]. In most patients, improvement of left ventricular function and regression of left ventricular hypertrophy[10] will occur. This process starts immediately after operation and may continue for decades after the surgical intervention[11]. It has been reported, that females show a better recovery of left ventricular function than males[12]. The lower transvalvular gradients associated with homografts and stentless valves[13] could result in a more complete regression of left ventricular hypertrophy than has been observed with mechanical prostheses or stented bioprostheses. Although some found a greater reduction of left ventricular mass in patients with a stentless valve compared to stented bioprosthesis[14], others were not able to confirm this finding[15,16]. Only large clinical trials comparing stented bioprosthetic valves, stentless bioprosthetic valves and mechanical valves in relation to survival, clinical status and regression of left ventricular hypertrophy will solve this issue.

Although regression of left ventricular hypertrophy is prominent in most patients after valve replacement, several factors can disturb this process: left ventricular mass is known to increase with age[17,18], with an even larger increase in females compared to males[19]. The presence of hypertension may inhibit complete regression of left ventricular hypertrophy.

AORTIC INSUFFICIENCY

Aortic insufficiency is associated with left ventricular volume overload. If aortic valve disease is not corrected, patients with aortic regurgitation follow a predictable course, which is characterized by progressive left ventricular dilation and left ventricular dysfunction[20]. In patients with compensated aortic insufficiency left ventricular end-diastolic volume, stroke volume and left ventricular mass will be increased, whereas left ventricular ejection fraction remains normal[2,12]. In patients with decompensated aortic insufficiency left ventricular end-diastolic volume, stroke volume and mass will be increased, whereas left ventricular ejection fraction remains normal[2,20]. The increase of left ventricular volume and mass is due to both parallel and series addition of new myofibrils in the ventricular myocardium[4]. After aortic valve replacement left ventricular dimension and left ventricular mass decreases in most patients within 6 months[21]. However, some patients will have persistent symptoms of congestive heart failure even if the after aortic valve has been replaced[22] These patients can be identified by a preoperative fractional shortening measured with echocardiography of less than 25%, an end-diastolic diameter greater than 38 mm/m^2 or an end-systolic dimension greater than 26 $mm/m^{2,21,23}$. These patients will fail to show any improvement in left ventricular function or decrease of left ventricular mass after aortic valve surgery.

OUR OWN EXPERIENCE IN PATIENTS WITH AORTIC VALVE DISEASE:

Our experience consists of the combined data-set of patients, who received a Freestyle stentless aortic bioprosthesis in Leiden, the Netherlands, Oxford, United Kingdom, Lille, France and Eindhoven, the Netherlands. Between June 1993 and June 1998, 240 patients, who received a Freestyle stentless bioprosthesis were echocardiographically examined 4 weeks after aortic valve replacement and 3-6 months, 1 year and 2 years after aortic valve replacement. Follow-up was complete in 167 patients after 3-6 months, 180 after 1 year and 108 after 2 years.

Mean age of the patient group was 68 years. Echocardiograms were made according to the guidelines proposed by the American Society of Echocardiography. Examinations included a M-Mode tracing, a two-dimensional echocardiogram in apical four and five chamber view, a pulsed Doppler recording of the left ventricular outflow velocities and a continuous wave Doppler recording of the aortic valve velocities. Additionally a color-flow Doppler image was performed from the parasternal long axis view and the apical view. Left ventricular mass was calculated using M-Mode measurements of wall thickness and left ventricular enddiastolic diameter according to the formula: Mass $= 1.04[(IVSd+LVDd+PWd)^3 - (LVDd)^3] -13.6$. In this formula IVSd = Interventricular septum at diastole, PWd = Posterior wall at diastole and LVDd = left ventricular dimension at diastole. Left ventricular volume was calculated according to the formula of Teichholz: Diastolic volume $= 7*(LVDd^3))/2.4 + LVDd)$. Shortening fraction was calculated as $(LVDd-LVDs)/LVDd * 100\%$.

In the present study, the mean gradient across the Freestyle xenograft was low: 7.9 ± 5.1 mmHg at discharge, decreasing to 5.5 mmHg after 3-6 months, 5.4 ± 3.7 mmHg after 1 year and 5.0 ± 3.5 mmHg after 2 years. The cardiac index was stable at 2.9 ± 1.0 l/min/m^2 throughout the study period. Aortic insufficiency grade 1 was present in 9.8% of the patients. In 0.9% of the patients it was grade 2. These patients had a paravalvular leackage. Left ventricular mass was 170.6 ± 72.3 g/m^2 within four weeks after valve replacement and had decreased to 143.6 ± 55.2 g/m^2 after 3-6 months, 135.6 ± 61.2 g/m^2 after 1 year and 133.5 ± 50.5 g/m^2 after 2 years (p<0.001). Left ventricular volume index remained stable and was 62.2 ± 30.2 ml/m^2 four weeks after surgery, 59.7 ± 24.5 ml/m^2 3-6 months after surgery, 62.9 ± 34.5 ml/m^2 1 year after surgery and 62.6 ± 20.9 ml/m^2 2 years after surgery.

Left ventricular ejection fraction increased from $54.2 \pm 17.7\%$ four weeks after operation to $58.6 \pm 15.4\%$ 3-6 months after surgery, $61.2 \pm 15.9\%$ one year after operation and $59.8 \pm 14.3\%$ two years after operation (p<0.001).

INFLUENCE OF ETIOLOGY ON LEFT VENTRICULAR REMODELING

We found different strata of left ventricular remodeling in patients with pure aortic stenosis, pure aortic insufficiency and combined aortic valve disease (Table 1-3).

Table 1. Hemodynamic and echocardiographic parameters in patients with Aortic Stenosis (AOS) during post operative follow-up of 2 years after valve replacement

AOS	< 4 weeks post surgery	3-6 months post surgery	1 year post surgery	2 years post surgery	
No of pts	161	108	123	72	
Mean valvular gradient (mmHg)	8.5 ± 5.4	5.4 ± 3.4	5.3 ± 3.8	5.4 ± 3.9	<0.0001
Cardiac Index (l/min/m2)	2.8 ± 0.9	2.8 ± 1.0	2.9 ± 0.9	2.9 ± 1.1	Ns
LVEDV index (ml/m2)	60.2 ± 26.6	60.4 ± 25.0	66.4 ± 39.3	57.6 ± 17.8	Ns
LV Mass Index (g/m2)	170.8± 66.8	144.8± 55.3	136.9 ± 67.7	122.0 ± 44.5	<0.0001
LVEF (%)	53.4 ± 18.1	58.7 ± 14.9	61.1 ± 16.0	61.6 ± 13.1	<0.0001

Table 2. Hemodynamic and echocardiographic parameters in patients with Aortic Insufficiency (AOI) during post operative follow-up of 2 years after valve replacement

AOI	< 4 weeks post surgery	3-6 months post surgery	1 year post surgery	2 years post surgery	P value
No of pts	44	21	21	18	
Mean valvular gradient	7.2 ± 4.4	3.4 ± 2.6	4.5 ± 3.4	5.1 ± 3.2	<0.0001
Cardiac Index	3.2 ± 1.3	3.1 ± 1.1	3.1 ± 0.9	3.2 ± 0.8	Ns
LVEDV index	76.6 ± 35.9	70.5 ± 24.7	65.1 ± 26.5	71.8 ± 26.6	Ns
LV Mass Index	196.7 ± 74.4	150.7 ± 60.3	145.7 ± 56.4	179.3 ± 63.1	<0.01
LVEF (%)	47.1 ± 20.4	52.2 ± 14.0	57.4 ± 15.8	62.1 ± 19.7	<0.05

Table 3. Hemodynamic and echocardiographic parameters in patients with AOS and AOI during post operative follow-up of 2 years after valve replacement

AOS/AOI	< 4 weeks post surgery	3-6 months post surgery	1 year post surgery	2 years post surgery	P value
No of pts	44	38	36	28	
Mean valvular gradient	6.0 ± 3.7	4.2 ± 2.4	4.5 ± 2.7	4.0 ± 2.7	< 0.005
Cardiac Index	2.9 ± 1.0	2.6 ± 0.7	2.7 ± 0.7	2.7 ± 0.9	Ns
LVEDV index	68.3 ± 33.1	68.5 ± 24.7	61.6 ± 23.4	64.9 ± 17.4	Ns
LV Mass Index	165.3 ± 67.7	139.2 ± 47.2	125.4 ± 54.5	128.2 ± 38.9	< 0.001
LVEF (%)	55.0 ± 14.9	56.9 ± 14.7	60.5 ± 14.8	56.7 ± 11.7	Ns

Table 4. Concommitant coronary artery disease and post operative hemodynamic and echocardiographic parameters during 2 year follow-up

	Coronary Artery Disease present < 4 weeks post surgery	Coronary Artery Disease absent < 4 weeks post surgery	Coronary Artery Disease present 2 years post surgery	Coronary Artery Disease absent 2 years post surgery	P value Presence versus Absence Coronary Artery Disease
Number of pts	94	161	53	72	
Mean valvular gradient	8.4 ± 5.3	7.4 ± 5.1	4.8 ± 2.7	5.1 ± 3.9	Ns
Cardiac Index	2.9 ± 1.0	2.8 ± 1.0	2.9 ± 0.9	2.9 ± 1.1	Ns
LVEDV index	63.1 ± 28.3	63.8 ± 31.7	65,1 ± 22,8	60.9 ± 19.1	Ns
LV Mass Index	184.3 ± 75.6	167.3 ± 68.5	144.8 ± 53.2	124.2 ± 46.1	<0.02
LVEF %	48.6 ± 19.9	58.7 ± 14.9	54.6 ± 16.8	61.2 ± 13.8	Ns

Pure aortic stenosis (a preoperative transvalvular gradient more than 50 mmHg without aortic insufficiency) was present in 67% of the patient population. Mean transvalvular gradient across the Freestyle valve was 8.5 ± 5.4 mmHg within four weeks after operation and decreased to 5.4 ± 3.9 mmHg two years after operation (p< 0.0001). Left ventricular ejection fraction was 53.4 ± 18.1 % within one month after operation and increased to 61.6 ± 13.0 % (p<0.0001). Left ventricular mass index was 170.8 ± 66.8 g/m^2 at discharge and decreased to 122.0 ± 44.5 g/m^2 after 2 years (p<0.0001). This meant a regression of left ventricular mass of 29%. It was obvious, that this patient group left ventricular function improved and left ventricular hypertrophy diminished considerably.

Pure aortic insufficiency (aortic insufficiency more than grade 2, without an increased transvalvular gradient) was present in 18% of patients. In these patients, mean postoperative transvalvular gradient across the Freestyle valve was 7.2 ± 4.4 mmHg and decreased to 4.9 ± 3.2 mmHg after two years (p<0.005). Left ventricular ejection fraction improved from $47.1 \pm 20.5\%$ to $60.9 \pm 19.6\%$ after two years (p<0.0001). Left ventricular mass index was higher early postoperative at 196 .7 ± 74.4 g/m^2 and showed a far less important decrease to 179.3 ± 63.1 g/m^2 after two years (P<0.01). Decrease of left ventricular hypertrophy was only 10% in this patient group. In 15% of the patients combined aortic valve disease (aortic stenosis and insufficiency) was present. In these patients the transvalvular gradient across the Freestyle valve was 6.0 ± 3.7 mmHg after operation and decreased to 4.0 ± 2.7 mmHg after 2 years (p< 0.001). Left ventricular ejection fraction was $55.0 \pm 14.9\%$ within some weeks after operation and remained the same ($56.7 \pm 11.7\%$) after 2 years. However, left ventricular mass index decreased to the same extend as was observed in patients with aortic stenosis, namely from 165.2 ± 67.7 g/m^2 to 128.2 ± 38.9 g/m^2 (p<0.01).

Despite the fact, that no complete information was available about left ventricular function before valve replacement, we can make the following conclusions:

Left ventricular mass decreases both in patients with aortic stenosis as in patients with aortic insufficiency. However, the extent of left ventricular remodeling is larger in patients with aortic stenosis. Recovery of left ventricular function can be observed both in patients with aortic stenosis and aortic insufficiency, but is absent in patients with combined aortic valve disease.

INFLUENCE OF CONCOMITANT CORONARY ARTERY DISEASE ON LEFT VENTRICULAR REMODELING

The influence of concomitant coronary artery disease on left ventricular remodeling can be observed in table 4. Patients with coronary artery disease, which was defined as a more than 50% stenosis in one of the epicardial coronary arteries showed equal transvalvular gradients, left ventricular ejection fraction and left ventricular volumes during two years follow-up. However, early postoperative left ventricular mass index was higher in patients with coronary artery disease and decreased less than in those patients who did not have significant coronary atherosclerosis (p<0.02). This is in agreement with the few data available on the consequence of coronary artery disease on the adaptation of the left ventricle to aortic stenosis. Patients with aortic stenosis and coronary artery disease have a higher systolic wall stress because of a less pronounced hypertrophy than patients with aortic stenosis and normal coronary arteries[24,25]. The negative effects of hypertrophy on left ventricular function would therefore appear earlier in the course of aortic stenosis if coronary artery disease is associated.

MITRAL INSUFFICIENCY

Mitral regurgitation burdens the left ventricle with an excessive volume load, that leads to a series of compensatory myocardial and circulatory adjustments[26,27].

Initially, volume overload is associated with an increase of left ventricular enddiastolic volume and left ventricular mass and preserved left ventricular contractility[28]. Because of the low impedance of the ejection into the left atrium afterload is reduced. This reduction in afterload allows end-systolic volume and ejection fraction to remain near-normal[29]. If severe mitral insufficiency persists, the left ventricle dilates considerably. The progressive left ventricular dilation increases systolic wall stress and end-systolic volume with a diminished left ventricular function[30,31]. Dilation of the mitral annulus results in a further increased severity of mitral insufficiency and progressive deterioration of left ventricular function. After some time left ventricular dysfunction becomes irreversible despite surgical correction of the mitral valve[32]. Preoperative left ventricular function has been identified as the most important predictor of postoperative outcome after mitral valve surgery[33].

In the clinical situation and in clinical studies, left ventricular function is frequently measured by left ventricular ejection fraction. However, left ventricular ejection fraction, is afterload dependent[34] and often remains higher than expected, thus masking the presence of left ventricular dysfunction[35]. Measurement of the maximal elastance at endsystole will reflect better left ventricular performance, because it is less dependent of changes in afterload[36]. After valve replacement left ventricular ejection fraction will often drop because of an increase in systolic wall stress[37].

Treatment of severe mitral insufficiency is beyond debate. Mitral valve repair is preferred because of the lower perioperative mortality and improved event-free late outcome. The treatment of moderate ischemic mitral regurgitation (grade 2) is a matter of debate. Normally, moderate mitral regurgitation is not corrected at the time of bypass surgery. However a subgroup analysis of SAVE (survival and ventricular enlargement trial) showed, that moderate mitral regurgitation has a negative prognostic outcome in patients with myocardial infarction[24]. Whether the correction of moderate ischemic mitral insufficiency by valve repair will improve outcome has to be determined by further studies.

Two groups of patients, who will perform differently after operation can be identified[37,38]
In the first group, preoperative echocardiographically measured left ventricular endsystolic dimension is lower than 26 mm/m^2 mm and left ventricular ejection shortening fraction is higher than 31%. In these patients, enddiastolic dimension and left ventricular mass decrease with a slight decrease in ejection fraction. In the second group with a severely enlarged left ventricle and a left ventricular endsystolic dimension more than 26 mm/m^2 or a left ventricular shortening fraction lower than 31%, left ventricular dimensions and mass do not fall. However, after operation, left ventricular ejection fraction drops dramatically in this group. In addition, these patients will remain symptomatic despite surgery. The advantages of an early operation in patients with severe mitral regurgitation are even more pronounced in patients who have concomitant coronary artery disease[39]. The association of

coronary lesions with severe mitral regurgitation should therefore an incentive to consider early valve repair.

Besides the preoperative myocardial status, mechanical integrity of the mitral apparatus appears to be another important factor in preservation of postoperative left ventricular function. Patients, whose mitral apparatus is left intact show minimal reduction in left ventricular ejection fraction, whereas patients in whom the mitral valve is completely excised show a significant reduction in postoperative left ventricular ejection fraction[40]. Therefore mitral valvuloplasty has been shown superiority to valve replacement for preservation of left ventricular function after mitral valve surgery[41].

REFERENCES

1. Kennedy J.W., Doces J., Stewart D.K.: Left ventricular function before and following aortic valve replacement. Circulation 1977; 56: 944-950.
2. Krayenbuehl H.P., Hess O.M., Monrad S., Schneider J., Mall G., Turina M. Left ventricular myocardial structure in aortic valve disease before, intermediate, and late after aortic valve replacement. Circulation 1989; 79: 744-755.
3. Schwarz F., Flameng W., Schaper J., Hehrlein F. Correlation between myocardial structure and diastolic properties of the heart in chronic aortic valve disease: Effects of corrective surgery. Am. J.Cardiol. 1976; 42: 895-903.
4. Grossman W. Cardiac hypertrophy: Useful adaptation or pathologic process? Am. J. Med. 1980; 69: 576-584.
5. Ross J. Jr. Afterload mismatch and preload reserve: a conceptual framework for the analysis of ventricular function. Prog. Cardiovasc. Dis. 1976; 18: 255-264.
6. Carroll J.D., Caroll E.P., Feldman T., Ward D.M., Lang R.M., McGaughy D., Karp R.B. Sex-associated differences in left ventricular function in aortic stenosis in the elderly. Circulation 1992; 86: 1099-1107.
7. Morris J.J., Schaff H.V., Mullany C.J., Rastogni A., McGregor C.G.A., Daly R.C., Frye R.L., Orszulak T.A. Determinants of survival and recovery of left ventricular function after aortic valve replacement. Ann. Thor. Surg. 1993; 56: 22-30.
8. Orsinelli D.A., AurigemmaG.P., Battista S., Krendel S., Gaasch W.H. Left ventricular hypertrophy and mortality after aortic valve replacement for aortic stenosis. J. Am. Coll. Cardiol. 1993; 22: 1679-1683.
9. Harpole D.H., Jones R.H. Serial assessment of ventricular performance after valve replacement for aortic stenosis. J. Thorac. Cardiovasc. Surg. 1990; 99: 645-650.
10. Pantely G., Morton M., Rahimtoola S.H. Severe aortic stenosis with impaired left ventricular function and clinical heart failure: results of valve replacement. Circulation 1978; 58: 255-264.
11. Monrad E.S., Hess O.M., Murakami T., Nonogi H., Corin W.J., Krayenbuel H.P. Abnormal exercise hemodynamics in patients with normal systolic function late after valve replacement. Circulation 1988; 77: 613-624.
12. Morris J.J., Schaff H.V., Mullany C.J., Morris P.B., Frye R.L., Orszulak T.A. Gender differences in left ventricular function response to aortic valve replacement. Circulation 1994; 90: [part 2]: II-183-II-189.
13. Baur L.H.B., J. Braun, C.H. Peels, A.P. Kappetein, Y. Houdas, A. Prat, B.H.M. van Straten, A. van de Ploeg, A. Sieders, P.J. Voogd, A.V.G. Bruschke, H.A. Huysmans. Haemodynamics of the Freestyle stentless aortic bioprosthesis. Cardiologie 1998; 5: 555-561.
14. Jin X.Y., Zhong Z.M., Gibson D.G., Yacoub M.H., Pepper J.R. Effects of valve substitute on changes in left ventricular function and hypertrophy after aortic valve replacement. Ann. Thorac. Cardiovasc. Surg. 1996; 62: 1084-1089.
15. Christakis G.T., Joyner C.D., Morgan C.D., Fremes S.E., Buth K.J., Sever J.Y., Rao V., Panagiotopoulos K.P., Murphy P.M., Goldman B.S. Left ventricular mass regression early after aortic valve replacement. Ann Thorac. Surg. 1996; 62: 1084-1089.
16. De Paulis R., Sommariva L., Colagrande L., De Matteis G.M., Fratini S., Tomai F., Bassano C., Penta de Peppo A., Chiariello L. Regression of left ventricular hypertrophy after aortic valve replacement for aortic stenosis with different valve substitutes. J. Thorac. Cardiovasc. Surg. 1998; 116: 590-598.
17. Messerli F.H., Clinical determinants and manifestations of left ventricular hypertrophy. In: Messerli F.H., ed. The heart and hypertension. New York: Yorke Medical Books; 1987; 219-230.

18. Lindroos M., Kupari M., Heikkila J., Tilvis R. Echocardiographic evidence of left ventricular hypertrophy in a general aged population. Am. J. Cardiol. 1994; 74: 385-390.
19. Shub C., Klein A.S., Zachariah P.K., Bailey K.R., Tajik A.J. Determination of left ventricular mass by echocardiography in a normal population: effect of age and sex in addition to body size. Mayo Clin. Proc. 1994; 69: 205-211.
20. Ross J. Afterload mismatch in aortic and mitral valve disease: Implications for surgical therapy. J.Am. Coll. Cardiol. 1985; 5: 811-826.
21. Henry W.L., Bonow R.O., Borer J.S, Kent K.M., Ware J.H., Redwood D.R., Itscoitz S.B., McIntosh C.L., Morrow A.G., Epstein S.E. Evaluation of aortic valve replacement in patients with valvular aortic stenosis. Circulation 1980; 61: 814-825.
22. Schuler G., Peterson K.L., Johnson A.D. Serial noninvasive assessment of left ventricular hypertrophy and function after surgical correction of aortic regurgitation. Am. J. Cardiol. 1979; 44: 585-594.
23. Gaasch W.H., Carroll J.D., Levine H.J., Criscitiello M.G. Chronic aortic regurgitation: prognostic value of the left ventricular end-diastolic and the end-systolic dimension and end-diastolic radius/thickness ratio. J. Am.Coll. Cardiol. 1983; 1: 775-782.
24. Iung B. Interface between valve disease and ischemic heart disease. Heart 2000; 84: 347-352.
25. Lund O., Flo C., Jensen FT Left ventricular systolic and diastolic function in aortic stenosis. Prognostic value after valve replacement and underlying mechanisms. Eur. Heart J. 1997; 18: 1977-1987
26. Gaasch W.H., Levine H.J., Zile M.R. Chronic aortic and mitral regurgitation: mechanical consequences of the lesion and the results of surgical correction. In: Gaasch W.H., Levine H.J., eds. The Ventricle. Boston: Martinus Nijhof Publishing, 1985; 237.
27. Carabello B.A. Mitral valve disease. Curr. Probl. Cardiol. 1993; 18: 421-480.
28. Eckberg D.L., Gault J.H., Bouchard R.L., Karliner J.S., Ross J. Jr. Mechanics of left ventricular contraction in chronic severe mitral regurgitation. Circulation 1973; 47: 1252-1259.
29. Wisenbaugh T., Spann J.F., Carabello B.A. Differences in myocardial performance and load between patients with similar amounts of chronic aortic versus chronic mitral regurgitation. J. Am. Coll. Cardiol. 1984; 3: 916-923.
30. Gaasch W.H., Zile M.R. Left ventricular function after surgical correction of chronic mitral regurgitation. Eur. Heart J. 12 (suppl B): 48-51, 1991.
31. Starling M.R., Kirsh M.M., Montgomery D.G., et al. Impaired left ventricular contractile function in patients with long-term mitral regurgitation and normal ejection fraction. J.Am. Coll.Cardiol. 22: 239-250, 1993.
32. Starling M.R. Effects of valve surgery on left ventricular contractile function in patients with long-term mitral regurgitation. Circulation 92; 811-818, 1995.
33. Enriquez-Sarano M., Schaff H.V., Orszulak T.A., et al Congestive heart failure after surgical correction of mitral regurgitation: A long-term study. Circulation 92: 2496- 2503, 1995.
34. Quinones M.A., Gaasch W.H., Alexander J.K. Influence of acute changes in preload, afterload contractile state and heart rate on ejection and isovolumic indices of myocardial contractility in man. Circulation 53: 293-302, 1976.
35. Wisenbaugh T. Does normal pump function belie muscle dysfunction in patients with chronic severe mitral regurgitation? Circulation 77: 515-525, 1988.
36. Kass DA, Maughan WL, et al. Comparative influence of load versus inotropic states on indexes of ventricular contractility: experimental and theoretical analysis based on P-V relationships. Circulation 1987;76:1422-1436.
37. Schuler G., Peterson K.L., Johnson A.D, Francis G., Dennish G., Utley J., Daily P.O., Ashburn W., Ross J. Jr. Temporal response of left ventricular performance to mitral valve surgery. Circulation 59: 1218-1231, 1979.
38. Zile M.R., Gaasch W.H., Carroll J.D., Levine H.J. Chronic mitral regurgitation: predictive value of preoperative echocardiographic indexes of left ventricular function and wall stress. J. Am. Coll. Cardiol. 1984; 3: 235-242.

39. Triboulloy C, Enriquez-Sarano M, Schaff HV. Impact of preoperative symptoms on survival after surgical correction of organic mitral regurgitation. Rationale for optimizing surgical indications. Circulation 1999; 99: 400-405.

40. David T.E., Uden D.E., Strauss H.D. The importance of the mitral apparatus in left ventricular function after correction of mitral regurgitation. Circulation 68: II-76-82, 1983.

41. Goldman M.E., Mora F., Guarino T., Fuster V., Mindlich B.P. Mitral valvuloplasty is superior to valve replacemnt for preservation of left ventricular function: An intraoperative two-dimensional echocardiographic study. J. Am. Coll. Cardiol. 10: 568-575, 1987.

VALVE PROSTHESIS - PATIENT MISMATCH
How to assess it and is it really a clinical problem?

Dr. R.B.A. VAN DEN BRINK, A.P. YAZDANBAKHSH, Prof.Dr. B.A.J.M. DE MOL

INTRODUCTION

Cardiac valve replacement has been a major advance for treatment of valvular heart disease during the past forty years.

Despite continuing improvements in design of prosthetic heart valves, devices used for valve replacement have not been perfect; so that in effect, the patient is exchanging one disease process for another. From the early days of valve replacement complications associated with valve replacement, such as primary structural dysfunction, thrombo-embolism, bleeding from anticoagulant therapy and endocarditis have received widespread attention.

In a classical paper in Circulation in 1978 Rahimtoola focussed attention on yet another problem with valve replacement devices namely: valve prosthesis-patient mismatch.[1]

Valve prosthesis - Patient Mismatch (VP-PM) can be considered to be present when the effective prosthetic valve area, after insertion into the patient, is less than that of a normal human valve. Accordingly, VP-PM is present in all prosthetic valves in which leaflets or occluder are suspended in a frame and sewing ring. This applies particularly for mechanical valves, and stented heterograft valves. The problem of VP-PM can be avoided by using stentless heterograft valves, homografts of adequate size or by aortic root enlargement.

Aim of the present paper is to discuss the assessment and clinical consequences of Valve Prosthesis - Patient Mismatch (VP-PM) after aortic valve replacement and mitral valve replacement.

ASSESSMENT OF VALVE PROSTHESIS - PATIENT MISMATCH (VP-PM)

The existence of Valve prosthesis- Patient Mismatch at the time of implantation may be determined by assessment of the prosthetic valve orifice area indexed for body surface area. The Prosthetic valve orifice area can be acquired by using

138

specifications of *primary* orifice area (*geometric* orifice area) that are supplied by the manufacturer. Prosthetic valve orifice area can also be derived from in vitro measurements on a pulse duplicator; this is called the *in vitro effective* orifice area. The effective prosthetic orifice area is often considerably smaller than the primary (geometric) prosthetic orifice area[2,3,4]. See figure 1A, 1B, 1C, 1D.

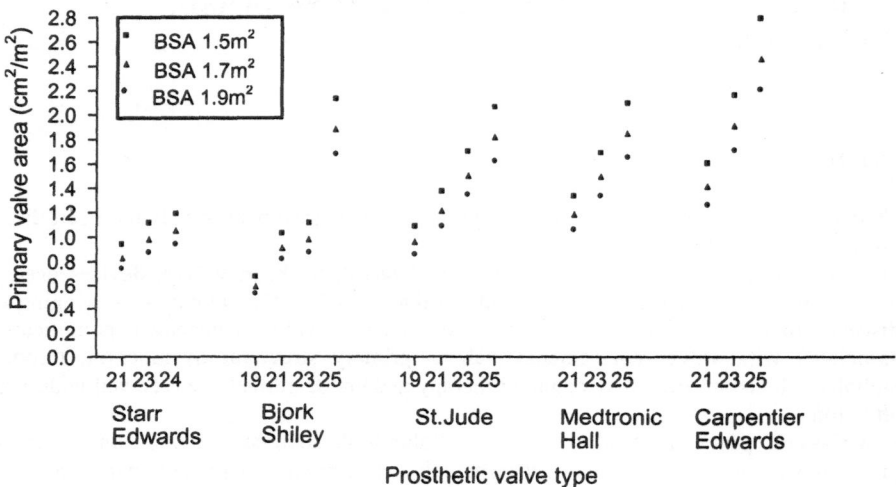

Figure 1A.: Different prosthetic valve types and sizes on the X-axis and the primary valve area of aortic prostheses corrected for body surface area on the Y-axis. Specifications of primary orifice area (geometric orifice area) are supplied by the manufacturer.

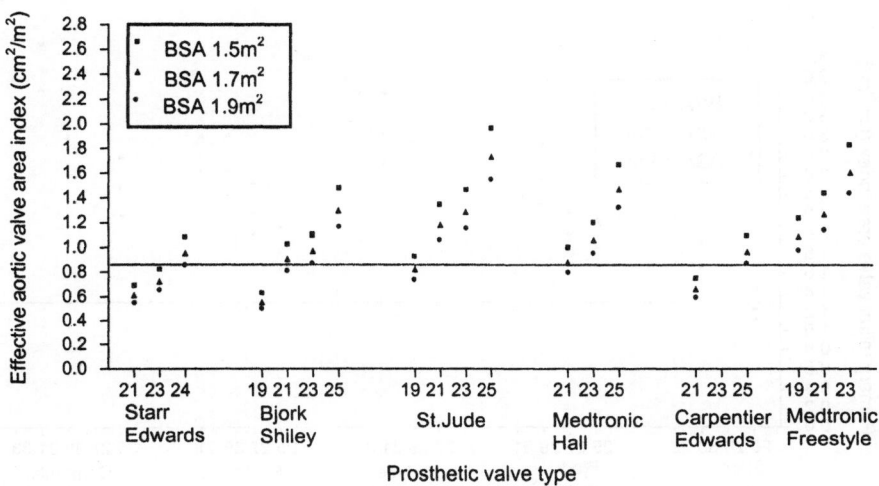

Figure 1B.: *Different prosthetic valve types and sizes on the X-axis and the in vitro effective valve area of aortic prostheses corrected for body surface area on the Y-axis.*

Horizontal line: In vitro experiments have shown that an effective prosthetic valve orifice area < 0.9 cm² / m² for aortic valve replacement was associated with an exponential increase in transprosthetic pressure gradients (Dumesnil, Yoghanathan). In literature this value is often used to indicate Valve Prosthesis–Patient mismatch.

Primary mitral valve area index (cm²/m²)

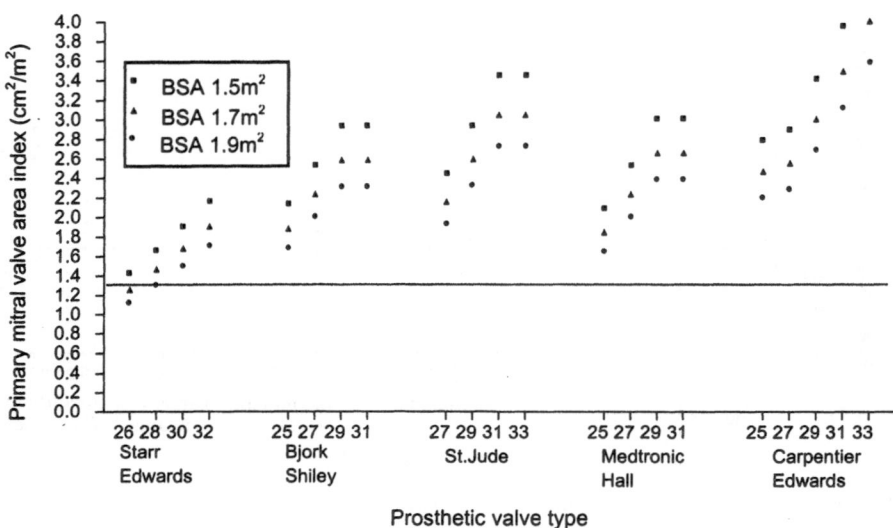

Figure 1C.: *Different prosthetic valve types and sizes on the X-axis and the primary valve area of mitral prostheses corrected for body surface area on the Y-axis. Specifications of primary orifice area (geometric orifice area) are supplied by the manufacturer. Observations in children with implanted mitral valve prostheses and in vitro studies indicate that for mitral valve prostheses the lower boundary for the occurrence of Valve Prosthesis- Patient mismatch might lie at a valve area index of ≤ 1.2 – 1.3 cm² /m² ; see horizontal line.*

Effective mitral valve area index (cm²/m²)

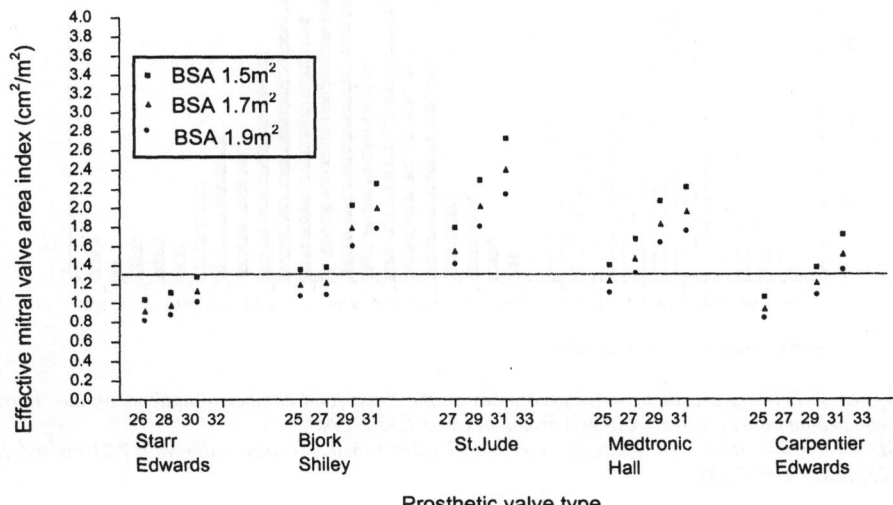

Figure 1D: *Different prosthetic valve types and sizes on the X-axis and the in vitro effective valve area of mitral prostheses corrected for body surface area on the Y-axis. Horizontal line: see legends to figure 1 C.*

The disadvantage of using effective prosthetic orifice area rather than primary (geometric) prosthetic orifice area is that values of the former may differ among laboratories even with the same cardiac output.

The primary prosthetic valve orifice area indexed for body surface area of patients who underwent aortic valve replacement (1980-1990) or mitral valve replacement (1980-1995) in our hospital is depicted in figure 2. The patients mainly received Björk Shiley, Medtronic Hall and St. Jude prosthetic valves. There is a normal distribution of the indexed primary prosthetic valve orifice areas in our patient population.

142

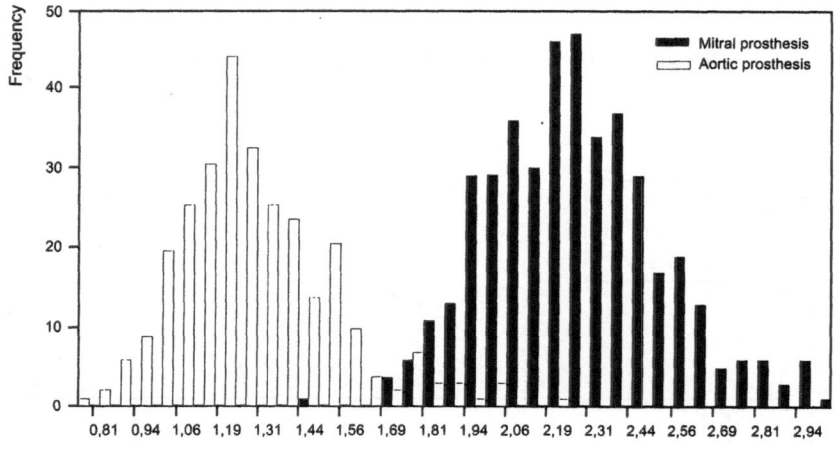

*Figure 2. Primary prosthetic valve area index on the X-axis and number of patients on the Y-axis . Mean primary aortic valve prosthesis area index was 1.33 cm²/m²
(SD 0.23; range 0.84-2.25. Mean primary mitral valve prosthesis area index was 2.21 cm²/m² (SD 0.23; range 1.36-3.18)*

The problem of VP-PM can be expected to occur in a patient with a large body surface area and a small annulus. A small annulus may be present in a patient with a stenotic valve lesion or an acute regurgitant lesion. In these patients pre-operative annulus diameter measurement is important. The annulus can be measured pre-operatively by two-dimensional echocardiography. The accuracy of transthoracic echocardiographic measurement of aortic annulus diameter is operator dependent, but is usually within 2 mm of intra-operative measurements with the surgical obturator[5] Trans-esophageal annulus measurement is somewhat more accurate in the prediction of prosthesis size than transthoracic echocardiography.[6]

Aortic valve prosthesis - patient mismatch

The adult human aortic valve area (AVA) is $3 - 4$ cm² or indexed to body surface area (average 1.75 m²) it is > 1.75 cm²/m². The native human aortic valve can be considered mildly stenotic if AVA is 1.5 - 3 cm² or $0.9 - 1.75$ cm²/m², moderately stenotic if AVA is 1 - 1.5 cm² or 0.6 - 0.9 cm²/m² and severely stenotic if AVA is < 0.8-1 cm² or $< 0.4 - 0.6$ cm²/m². [7,8] It is generally accepted that native aortic valve stenosis is clinically relevant if the indexed valve area is $\leq 0.85 - 0.9$ cm²/m².

Based on the aforementioned values for native aortic valves, aortic valve prosthesis – patient mismatch (AVP-PM) has been defined as follows: mild AVP-PM is said to be present if effective prosthetic orifice area is $0.9 - 1.75$ cm²/m², moderate AVP-PM if it is $0.6 - 0.9$ cm²/m², and severe AVP-PM exists if the effective prosthetic valve area index is ≤ 0.6 cm²/m². [5]

Dumesnil and Yoghanathan demonstrated that an effective prosthetic valve orifice area < 0.9 cm²/m² for aortic valve replacement was associated with an exponential increase in transprosthetic pressure gradients[9].

In vitro effective prosthetic valve orifice areas have been determined for all prosthetic valve types and sizes with pulse duplicators. Using these figures one can calculate the in vitro effective orifice area of prosthetic valves indexed to body surface area for an individual patient at the time of implantation; See figure 1B.

Especially, size 19 mm Starr Edwards and Björk Shiley valves are within the range of severe AVP-PM (≤ 0.6 cm²/m²), when they are inserted in normal sized adults (Body Surface Area > 1.7 m²). Moderate AVP-PM (≤ 0.9 cm²/m²) is present if St. Jude Standard size 19, Starr Edwards size 19 and 21, Björk- Shiley size 19 and 21 or Carpentier Edwards bioprostheses size 19 and 21 are used. Medtronic Freestyle (stentless) valves only show mild AVP-PM, even if a size 19 is implanted in an individual with a BSA of 1.9 m².

In our own cohort of 171 patients with Björk Shiley valves severe AVP-PM (effective orifice area ≤ 0.6 cm²/m²) was present in 2 % and moderate AVP-PM (≤ 0.85 cm²/m²) in 45 %.

Mitral valve prosthesis – patient mismatch (mvp-pm)

The adult human mitral valve area (MVA) is 4 - 5 cm² or indexed to body surface area it is > 2.3 cm²/m². The native human mitral valve can be considered mildly stenotic if MVA is 1.5 - 2.5 cm² or 0.9 - 1.5 cm²/m², moderately stenotic if MVA is 1-1.5 cm² or 0.6 - 0.9 cm²/m² and severely stenotic if MVA is < 1 cm² or < 0.6 cm²/m². Patients with native mitral valve stenosis are considered to have clinically relevant stenosis if the indexed valve area is ≤ 0.9 cm²/m². [4,5]

Figure 1 C shows the primary prosthetic valve orifice area index for different types of mitral prostheses. Specifications of primary orifice area (geometric orifice area) can be obtained from the manufacturer.

Dumesnil and Yoghanathan [6] using an in vitro pulse duplicator demonstrated that an effective prosthetic valve orifice area < 1.3 cm²/m² for mitral valve replacement was associated with an exponential increase in transprosthetic pressure gradients. In vitro effective prosthetic valve orifice areas have been determined for all prosthetic valve types and sizes with pulse duplicators. Using these figures one can calculate the in vitro effective orifice area of prosthetic valves indexed to body surface area for an individual patient at the time of implantation; See figure 1D.

CLINICAL IMPACT OF VALVE PROSTHESIS - PATIENT MISMATCH

Clinical impact of aortic valve prosthesis – patient mismatch (avp-pm)

Few studies focussed on the mortality and morbidity of AVP-PM using the prosthetic valve area at the time of implantation corrected for body surface area. See table 1.

Table 1. Clinical impact of Aortic Valve Prosthesis- Patient mismatch. Studies using Primary (geometric) prosthetic orifice area index [&] or Effective prosthetic orifice area index [*] to define the extent of mismatch

	Pibarot[10][*]	Pibarot[11][*]	Fernandez[12][&]
Number	329	61	607
Period	1986-1995	1991-1992	1982-1991
Age	70±9/67±9[^]	73± 10	59.8
			(8.89)
Prosthesis	Medtronic Intact Bioprosthesis	Bioprothesis[**]	St.Jude Medical
CABG (%)	33	41	30
VAI (cm²/m²)	$\leq$0.85 (46%)	$\leq$0.85 (52%)	1.31
	> 0.85 (54%)	> 0.86 (48%)	(0.74-2.86)
Follow-Up (yrs)	7	6.2 ± 4.4	2.7
Endpoint	Early mort. (NS)	NYHA III/IV (NS)	Early mort. (NS)
	Late mort. (NS)	Syncope (p=0.05)	Late mort. (NS)
	NYHA class (p=0.009)[#]	AP (p=0.27)	NYHA class (NS)
		Pulm.Edema (p=0.46)	Valve-related Events[***] (NS)

&   *Geometric (or primary) prosthetic orifice area supplied by the manufacturer divided by the patient's body surface area.*

*   *Effective prosthetic orifice area determined in vitro with a pulse duplicator*

^   *VAI ≤ 0.85 cm²/m² respectively > 0.85 cm²/m²*

\#   *Less improvement of functional class in mismatch group (VAI≤ 0.85 cm²/m²)*

**   *Baxter Edward, Medtronic, Hancock (and 5 St. Jude Medical)*

***   *Valve-related events: major thromboembolism, anticoagulant related hemorrhage or reoperation*

CABG= coronary bypass grafting; VAI= prosthetic valve orifice area index (cm²/m² BSA); BSA=body surface area

Pibarot et al[10] examined 329 adult patients who underwent aortic valve replacement with Medtronic Intact aortic bioprostheses, of whom 33 % had concurrent Coronary Artery Bypass Grafting (CABG); mean follow-up was 7 years. The in vitro effective orifice area divided by the patient's body surface area were used as a measure of AVP-PM. Severe AVP-PM (≤ 0.6 cm^2/m^2) was present in 3 % of his population and moderate AVP-PM (≤ 0.85 cm^2/m^2) in 43 %. In this study AVP-PM (effective orifice area ≤ 0.85 cm^2/m^2) had no significant impact both on patient survival (75 ± 4% and 79 ± 3%, respectively) and on valve-related morbidity. However, AVP-PM was associated with significantly less post-operative improvement of the functional class according to the NYHA classification (p=0.009) and congestive heart failure at 5 years was significantly more common in those with AVP-PM (15± 3% vs. 7 ± 4%; p=0.05). In a subgroup of 61 prospectively included patients[11], who received a bioprosthesis and who underwent a post-operative Dopplerechocardiographic examination they found after a mean follow-up of 6.2 ± 4.4 years a significantly higher number of adverse clinical events (50% vs.21%; p=0.017). See table 1. Clinical events in that study were defined as a history of syncopal events, angina pectoris and /or acute pulmonary oedema after valve implantation. The difference between groups was mainly caused by syncopal events. Pre-operative predictors of AVP-PM were: larger body surface area (BSA), older age and native valve stenosis.[10, 11]

Fernandez et al[12] investigated 607 adult patients who underwent aortic valve replacement with St. Jude Medical valves, of whom 30% had concomitant CABG or valve repair (7%); mean follow-up was 2.7 years. The primary orifice area divided by the patient's body surface area was used as a measure of AVP-PM. Mean prosthetic valve area index was 1.31 cm^2 / m^2 (0.74-2.86 cm^2/m^2). In this study prosthetic valve area index was tested as a continuous variable; it was not an independent risk factor for early death, late death, NYHA class or valve-related events (major thrombo-embolism, anticoagulant related haemorrhage or reoperation).

Three studies on the mortality and morbidity of AVP-PM used Body Surface Area combined with valve size (diameter) as a measure for mismatch. See table 2.

He et al[13] reported on survival after aortic valve replacement in a cohort of 447 patients with small sized prostheses (21 mm or less) of whom 26% underwent concomitant CABG; mean follow-up was 7.1 ± 6.4 years. Prosthetic valves used were mainly Starr Edwards, Carpentier Edwards porcine and 41 St. Jude Medical standard. Mean BSA was 1.69 ± 0.18 m^2 (range 1.06 to 2.23 m^2), BSA was less than 1.7 m^2 in 150 patients. In this study eleven variables among which BSA as a continuous variable and small BSA (less than 1.6, 1.7, 1.8 or 1.9 m^2), were investigated with regard to long-term survival. In the subgroup of patients with concomitant CABG, a BSA less than 1.7 m^2 was the only independent predictor for long-term survival. In other words: mismatch between body size and prosthesis size was a negative determinant for long-term survival only in patients with concomitant CABG. They suggested that the influence of AVP-PM in the subgroup with CAGB might have been more obvious because of impaired cardiac reserve and because in most of these patients the primary indication for operation had been coronary artery disease rather than the severity of the aortic valve lesion.

Table 2. Clinical impact of Aortic Valve Prosthesis- Patient mismatch
Studies using valve size related to body surface area [&] to define the extent of mismatch

	He[13]	Sawant[14]	Kratz[15]
Number	447	327	254
Period	1961-1993	1978-1994	1979-1990
Age	65.5 ± 14.5	64 ± 11	54 ± 15
Prosthesis type	Starr Edwards Carpentier Edwards St. Jude Medical	St.Jude Medical	St.Jude Medical
Prosthesis size	≤ 21	≤ 21	≤ 21
CABG (%)	26	33	25
BSA (m^2)	≤ 1.7 in 34% 1.7-1.9 in 66% ≥ 1.9 in 34%	< 1.9 in 78% ≥ 1.9 in 22%	≤ 1.7 in 71% 1.7-1.9 in 18 % ≥ 1.9 in 11%
BSA mean (m^2)	1.69 ± 0.18	1.7 ± 0.27	
(range)	(1.06 - 2.23)	(1.20 – 2.26)	(1.30 – 2.6)
Follow-Up (yrs)	7.1 ± 6.4	6.2 ± 3.9	4.4 ± 3.1
Endpoint	Long-term survival In AVR+CABG group BSA ≤ 1.7 m^2 (p=0.014)	Long-term survival (NS)	All cause late mort (NS) Sudden death (p=0.0095)* Death due to CHF (NS)

CHF=Congestive Heart Failure
* In the subgroup with BSA > 1.9m^2

Sawant et al[14] investigated 327 patients who underwent aortic valve replacement with a small prosthesis (≤ 21 mm) of whom 33 % underwent concomitant CABG; mean follow-up was 6.2 ± 3.9 years and mean BSA was 1.7 ± 0.27 m^2 (range 1.20 to 2.26 m^2), BSA was ≥ 1.9 m^2 in 58 patients (22%). They investigated the impact of 5 variables, among which BSA as a continuous variable, on long-term mortality and valve-related morbidity and found that BSA was no independent predictor.

A cohort of 254 adult patients with small (19 or 21 mm) St. Jude aortic valve prostheses was investigated by Kratz et al[15]; 25% underwent concomitant CABG; mean follow-up was 4.4 ± 3.1; BSA was > 1.7 m^2 in 69 patients (27%) and BSA was > 1.9 m^2 in 27 patients (11%). They found that a BSA >1.7 m^2 and even a BSA > 1.9 m^2 was no independent risk factor for all cause late death or late death associated with congestive heart failure. In the group with BSA > 1.9 m^2 there was an increased risk for late sudden death (p=0.0095).

Hirooka et al[16] demonstrated that the geometric valve area index correlated with peak oxygen consumption in a cohort of patients with St. Jude Medical valves at a mean of 2.2 years after valve replacement. They suggested that the geometric aortic prosthetic valve area index should be at least 1.5 cm^2/m^2 to achieve a good exercise capacity post-operatively (>80% of predicted peak oxygen consumption).

Several studies indicate that regression of ventricular hypertrophy is less in patients with small prosthetic valves (especially size 19 aortic prostheses in adults)[17,18] However, one other investigation in bi-leaflet aortic prostheses showed no significant influence of size on the pattern and extent of regression of left ventricular hypertrophy after an intermediate period of follow-up[19] In a randomized study Maselli et al. demonstrated that when a stentless valve or homograft aortic valve was used instead of a stented valve to replace a stenotic aortic valve, there was more complete or at least faster regression of left ventricular hypertrophy[20] As far as we know the impact of residual ventricular hypertrophy on outcome in patients after valve replacement has not been studied.
Although intuitively aortic valve prosthesis-patient mismatch should have an impact on mortality and morbidity, the aforementioned studies were rather equivocal. This could be due to the fact that most studies used BSA related to valve size rather than prosthetic valve orifice area indexed for body surface area as a measure for AVP-PM. Unfortunately manufacturers' labeling of valves is nonuniform and does not correspond to the internal diameters of the valves[21] Other reasons that clinical studies showed no impact of AVP-PM on mortality or morbidity may be that most of aforementioned studies did not analyze geometric valve area index as a continuous variable. It could be that follow-up was not long enough or that severe AVP-PM is rare and that moderate APV-PM produces no important clinical problems.
Yet another possibility is that prosthetic valve area indexed for BSA as the only measure for AVP-PM is a too limited way to investigate the impact of the size of a certain prosthetic valve type on outcome.
After all, the workload that is placed on the heart by a prosthetic valve is not only dependent on orifice area but it is also influenced by anatomic patient-related factors that lead to energy loss. These additional factors are the geometry of the inlet of the prosthetic valve (i.e. left ventricular outflow tract), the geometry of the outlet of the prosthetic valve (aortic root and ascending aorta) and the leakage volume of the prosthesis.[22]

CLINICAL IMPACT OF MITRAL VALVE PROSTHESIS – PATIENT MISMATCH (MVP-PM)

In the late seventies Rahimtoola described examples of probable mitral valve prosthesis - patient mismatch (MVP-PM) in adult patients.[1,23]

In 1990, we examined a young man of 18 years, who had received a Björk Shiley mitral prosthesis size 21 mm at his 7th year. At that time his BSA was 0.85 m^2 and the primary prosthetic valve area index was 1.8 cm^2/m^2. However, at his 18th year he became severely symptomatic. His BSA had increased to 1.73 m^2 and consequently the primary prosthetic valve area index had dropped to 0.89 cm^2 / m^2 , the mean transprosthetic gradient at rest was 17 mmHg. Reoperation showed no pannus. A St. Jude Medical prosthesis size 25 mm was inserted (primary prosthetic valve area index 1.86 cm^2/m^2). After this procedure the mean transprosthetic gradient dropped to 6 mmHg and his complaints of dyspnea disappeared.

Only few studies have been directed at the potentially deleterious effect of MVP-PM on the survival of patients after mitral valve replacement. See Table 3.

Fernandez et al.[12] investigated 539 adult patients who underwent mitral valve replacement with St. Jude Medical valves, of whom 13% had concomitant CABG or valve repair (14%); mean follow-up was 3.4 years. Mean primary prosthetic valve area index was 2.25 cm^2/m^2 (1.42-6.33 cm^2/m^2). In this study prosthetic valve area index was tested as a continuous variable; it was not an independent risk factor for early death, late death, NYHA class or valve-related events (major thromboembolism, anticoagulant related hemorrhage or reoperation).

Recently we performed a study to determine the role of mitral valve prosthesis – patient mismatch on survival in a cohort of consecutive patients after mitral valve replacement with a mechanical prosthesis, focussing on the lower tail of the normal distribution curve of the primary prosthetic valve area index (VAI)[24]. Our study population consisted of 428 adult patients who underwent mitral valve replacement by a Medtronic-Hall (n= 270, 63%) or a St Jude Medical prosthesis (n=158, 37%); 19% had concomitant CABG or valve repair (6%); mean age was 61.7±11.2 years and mean follow-up was 5.7 years. The valve area index showed a normal distribution curve ranging from 1.43 cm^2/m^2 to 2.98 cm^2/m^2 with a mean of 2.2 cm^2/m^2. The cut-off value of the 10th -percentile of the primary valve area index was 1.919 cm^2/m^2. Multivariate logistic regression analysis of the determinants of the 30-day mortality rendered a small primary valve area index (<1.9 cm^2/m^2) as an independent risk indicator: relative risk 4.27 (95% CI. 1.61 – 9.49; P=0.0043). The main death cause in this group was congestive heart failure. The overall 5 year survival between the two groups was significantly different (group 1 vs. group 2: 65.3% vs. 78.0% P= 0.037), but this difference was entirely due to the inclusion of the 30-day mortality.

Table 3. Clinical impact of Mitral Valve Prosthesis - Patient mismatch. Studies using primary prosthetic valve orifice area [&] to define the extent of mismatch

	Fernandez[12]		Yazdanbakhsh[24]
Number	539		428
Period	1982 - 1991		1980 – 1995
Age	55.8		61.7 ± 11.2
	(1-84)		(22-83)
Prosthesis	St.Jude Medical		St.Jude Medical
			Medtronic Hall
CABG (%)	13		19
Tricuspid valve repair (%)	14		6
VAI (cm^2/m^2)	2.55*		2.2
	(1.42-6.33)		(1.43-2.98)
			< 1.9 in 6%[#]
Follow-Up (yrs)	3.4		5.7
Endpoint	Early mort	(NS)	Early mort (p=0.005)
	Late mort	(NS)	RR 4.3 (95% CI:1.6-9.5)
	NYHA Class	(NS)	Late mort[$] (NS)
	Valve related		
	Events^	(NS)	

&   *Geometric prosthetic valve orifice area supplied by the manufacturer*
    CABG=coronary bypass grafting; VAI=prosthetic valve orifice area index; BSA=body surface area
*   *VAI tested as a continuous variable*
\#   *VAI tested as a dichotomous variable; Cut-off point of the 10th-percentile of the VAI was 1.919 cm^2/m^2.*
^   *Valve-related events: major thromboembolism, anticoagulant related hemorrhage or reoperation*
$ *Excluding early mortality*

The discrepancy of our results[24] with those of Fernandez et al.[12] may be due to the different distribution of body surface area of the patients in the latter study with an age range from 1 to 84 years, or to the fact that the lower tail of the distribution of VAI was not specifically addressed by Fernandez et al., to unknown confounding factors, or it may be due to chance. The causes of early death in our series give some support to the theory that extreme valve prosthesis– patient mismatch may cause heart failure in the early post-operative phase. Theoretically, this might be attributed to the combination of a persisting relatively high afterload of the right ventricle after implantation of a narrow prosthetic valve and stunning of the right ventricle in the early post-operative phase. It is conceivable that the correlation between narrow valves and early death, even if real, is not entirely causal. There may be hidden causes why surgeons prefer small valves in patients who have a bad prognosis. However, the effect remained after adjusting for possible confounders and the high significance of this relation means that any such hypothetical unknown confounder would have to be of similar force and highly correlated with small VAI to explain it.

In children re-replacement of mitral valve prosthesis because of somatic growth leading to valve prosthesis – patient mismatch is a well-known problem, especially if the child has been operated upon at a young age because of a parachute mitral valve complex. Unfortunately, in studies addressing this subject it is not documented at which level of valve area index, signs of heart failure develop.[25,26,27] However, from two reported studies and our own experience it may be inferred that severe heart failure leading to re-replacement of the prosthetic valve occurs at a primary mitral valve area index of $\leq$ 1.2 cm^2/m^2.[28,29]

The VAI of patients surviving the first 30 days in our population ranged from 1.67 cm^2/m^2 to 2.97 cm^2/m^2 (mean 2.25 cm^2/m^2), which was well above the aforementioned value of 1.2 cm^2/m^2. This might explain why the late mortality between the 30-day survivors in group 1 and group 2 in our study population was not significantly different.

CONCLUSION

Intuitively, there must be valve sizes that severely impair cardiac function, but general surgical practice may largely avoid this. Where exactly the permissible lower boundary of the primary prosthetic valve area index lies is hard to determine in adults. Observations in children with implanted **mitral valve prostheses** and in vitro studies indicate that for mitral valve prostheses it might lie at a primary valve area index of $\leq$ 1.2 – 1.3 cm^2/m^2. The most frequently implanted valve sizes in adults result in a primary mitral prosthesis valve area index of > 1.4 cm^2/m^2, which is well above the permissible lower boundary for Mitral valve prosthesis-Patient mismatch. This might be the reason that mitral valve prosthesis-patient mismatch has not yet turned out to be an important problem in clinical practice as far as medium-term mortality and morbidity is concerned (follow-up in published studies is 2 – 7 years). However, in the early post-operative phase the permissible lower boundary for mitral valve prosthesis-patient mismatch seems to lay somewhat higher (primary orifice area of 1.9 cm^2/m^2)[24].

For **aortic prostheses** the lower limit at which Aortic valve prosthesis - Patient mismatch occurs is even harder to determine as we have no examples of children who outgrow their prosthetic valve (aortic valve replacement in children usually can be delayed until an adult-sized valve prosthesis can be inserted). However, in vitro studies of aortic prosthetic valves show an exponential increase of transprosthetic gradient at an effective prosthetic valve area below 0.9 cm^2/m^2. One study suggested that the primary aortic prosthetic orifice area index should be at least 1.5 cm^2/m^2 to achieve a good exercise capacity post-operatively (i.e. >80% of predicted peak oxygen consumption).

The occurrence of VP-PM should especially be anticipated in large patients with a stenotic valve lesion or acute regurgitant lesion. In those patients the annulus diameter should be determined pre-operatively so that the cardiac surgeon is able to choose the optimal prosthetic valve (for example a stentless bioprosthesis or homograft) or adapt the surgical procedure (for example aortic root enlargement).

From a clinical point of view it is important to prevent VP-PM as this leads to better a better exercise capacity and to more complete regression of ventricular hypertrophy after valve replacement. Prevention of VP- PM in some studies also seems to improve survival and reduce the incidence of congestive heart failure.

REFERENCES

1. Rahimtoola SH. The problem of valve prosthesis-patient mismatch. Circulation 1978; 58: 20-24.
2. Walker DK, Scotten LN. A database obtained from in vitro function testing of mechanical heart valves. J Heart Valve Dis 1994; 3: 561-70.
3. Rashtian MY, Stevenson DM, Allen DT, Yoghanatan AP, Harrison EC, Edmiston WA, Faughan P, Rahimtoola SH. Flow characteristics of four commonly used mechanical valves. Am J Cardiol 1986; 58: 743-52.
4. Rashtian MY, Stevenson DM, Allen DT, Yoghanathan AP, Harrison EC, Edmiston WA, Rahimtoola SH. Flow characteristics of bioprosthetic heart valves. Chest 1990; 98: 365-75.
5. Greaves SC, Reimold CS, Lee RT, Cooke KA, Aranki SF. Preoperative prediction of prosthetic aortic valve annulus diameter by two-dimensional echocardiography. J Heart valve Dis 1995; 4: 14-17.
6. Abraham TP, Kon ND, Nomeir AM, Cordell AR, Kitzman DW. Accuracy of transesophageal echocardiography in preoperative determination of aortic annulus size during valve replacement. J Am Soc Echocardiogr 1997; 10: 149-154.
7. Bonow RO, Carabello B, de Leon AC, Edmunds LH, Fedderly BJ, Freed MD, Gaasch WH, McKay CR, Nishimura RA O'Gara PT, O'Rourke RA, Rahimtoola SH. ACC/AHA guidelines for the management of patients with valvular heart disease: a report of the American College of Cardiology/ American Heart
8. Association Task Force on pPractice guidelines. J Am Coll Cardiol 1998; 32: 1486-1588.
9. Rahimtoola SH,. Editorial: Valve prosthesis-Patient mismatch: an update. J Heart Valve Dis 1998; 7: 207-210
10. Dumesnil JG, Yoganathan AP. Valve prosthesis hemodynamics and the problem of high transprosthetic gradients. Eur J Cardiothorac Surg 1992; 6 (suppl 1): S34 – S38
11. Pibarot P, Dumesnil JG, Lemieux M, Cartier P, Metras J, Durand LG. Impact of prosthesis-patient mismatch on hemodynamic and symptomatic status, morbidity and mortality after aortic valve replacement with a bioprosthetic heart valve J Heart Valve Dis 1998; 7: 211-18
12. Pibarot P, Honos GN, Durand LG, Dumesnil JG. The effect of prosthesis-patient mismatch on aortic bioprosthetic valve hemodynamic performance and patient clinical status. Can J Cardiol 1996; 12: 379-87.
13. Fernandez J, Chen Ch, Laub G, Anderson WA, Brdlik OB, Murphy MM, McGrath LB. Predictive value of prosthetic valve area index for early and late clinical results after valve replacement with the St. Jude Medical valve prosthesis. Circulation 1996; 94 (suppl II): II-109 – II-112.
14. He GW, Grunkemeier GL, Gately HL, Furnary AP, Starr A. Up to thirthy-year survival after aortic valve replacement in the small aortic root. Ann Thorac Surg 1995; 59: 1056-62.
15. Sawant D, Singh AK, Feng WC, Bert AA, Rotenberg F. St. Jude Medical cardiac valves in small aortic roots: follow-up to sixteen years. J Thorac Cardiovasc Surg 1997; 113: 499-509.
16. Kratz JM, Sade RM, Crawford FA, Crumbley III AJ, Stroud MR. The risk of small St. Jude aortic valve prostheses. Ann Thorac Surg 1994;57:1114-9
17. Hirooka K, Kawazoe K, Kosakai Y, Sasako Y, Eishi K, Kito Y, Nakanishi N, Yoshioka T, Kawashima Y Prediction of postoperative exercise tolerance after aortic valve replacement. Ann Thorac Surg 1994; 58: 1626-1630.

18. Gonzalez-Juanatey JR, Garcia-Acuna JM, Fernandez MV, Cendon AA, Fuentes VC, Garci-Bengoechea JB, Gil de la Pena M. Influence of the size of aortic valve prostheses on hemodynamics and change in left ventricular mass: implications for the surgical management of aortic stenosis. J Thorac Cardiovasc Surg 1996; 112: 273-280.

19. Sim EKW, Orszulak TA, Schaff HV, Shub C. Influence of prosthesis size on change in left ventricular mass following aortic valve replacement. Eur J Cardiothorac Surg 1994; 8: 293-297.

20. De Paulis R, Sommariva L, De Matteis GM, Caprara E, Tomai F, Penta de Peppo A, Pollisca P, Bassano C, Chiariello L. Extent and pattern of regression of left ventricular hypertrophy in patients with small size carbomedics aortic valves. J Thorac Cardiovasc Surg 1997; 113: 901-909

21. Maselli D, Pizio R, Bruno LP, Di Bella I, De Gasperis C. Left ventricular mass reduction after aortic valve replacement: homografts, stentless and stented valves. Ann Thorac Surg 1999; 67: 966-71.

22. Christakis GT, Buth KJ, Goldman BS, Fremes SE, Rao V, Cohen C, Borger MA, Weisel RD. Inaccurate and misleading valve sizing: a proposed standard for valve size nomenclature. Ann Thorac Surg 1998; 66:1198-203.

23. Travis BR, Heinrich RS, Ensley AE, Gibson DE, Hashim S, Yoganathan AP. The hemodynamic effects of mechanical prosthetic valve type and orientation on fluid mechanical energy loss and pressure drop in in vitro models of ventricular hypertrophy. J Heart Valve Dis. 1998; 7: 345-54.

24. Rahimtoola SH, Murphy E. Valve prosthesis-patient mismatch. A long-term sequela. British Heart J 1981; 45: 331-335

25. Yazdanbakhsh AP, van den Brink RBA, Dekker E, de Mol BAJM. Small valve area index: its influence on early mortality after mitral valve replacement. Eur J Cardiothorac Surg 00 (2000) 1-6

26. Nudelman I, Schachner A, Levy MJ. Repeated mitral valve replacement in the growing child with congenital mitral valve disease. J Thorac Cardiovasc Surg 1980; 79: 765-769.

27. Lubiszewska B, Rozanski J, Szufladowicz M, Hoffman P, Ksiezycka E, Rydlewska-sadowska W, Ruzyllo W. Mechanical valve replacement in congenital heart disease in children. J Heart Valve Dis 1999; 8: 74-79.

28. Milano A, Vouché PR, Baillot-Vernant F, Donzeau-Gouge P, Trinquet F, Roux PM, Leca F, Neveux JY. Late results after left-sided cardiac valve replacement in children. J Thorac Cardiovasc Surg 1986; 92: 218-225.

29. Friedman S, Edmunds LH, Cuaso CC. Long-term mitral valve replacement in young children. Circulation 1978; 57: 981-986

30. Schaff HV, Danielson GK, Didonato RM, Puga JF, Mair DD, Mc Goon DC. Late results after Starr-Edwards valve replacement in children. J Thorac Cardiovasc Surg 1984; 88: 583-589

Section V / Chapter 1

VALVULAR HEART DISEASE:
IS IT EVER TOO LATE TO OPERATE?

C.H. PEELS

INTRODUCTION

When the decision is taken not to operate in a patient with valvular heart disease, the risk and prognosis direct peri- and postoperatively outweigh the clinical benefit and improvement in long-term prognosis after surgery.

Arguments to defer from operation can be on one hand the expectation that the removal of the valve lesion will not improve the clinical status of the patient anymore, an argument mostly caused by the dysfunction of the left ventricle ("cardiac" arguments). On the other hand, arguments to defer from operation can be non-cardiac for example comorbidity which makes the risk of operation too high.

Firstly, the cardiac arguments will be discussed for each of the often encountered valve lesions in adult cardiac surgery, thereafter the factors which create the comorbidity will be discussed.

A combination of these arguments is most of the time at stake and the risk of the surgical procedure must always be individually weighed against the potential benefit for the patient.

CARDIAC ARGUMENTS :
SEVERE AORTIC STENOSIS, WHEN NOT TOO OPERATE?

As discussed elsewhere in this course, the natural history and prognosis of patients with an asymptomatic severe valvular aortic stenosis has been well documented and survival resembles that of age and gender matched control subjects[1]. However, the occurrence of a cardiac event in the first 2 years is high, around 25%, and one should follow these patients closely and intervene when symptoms occur.

When this optimal moment for surgical intervention is missed or a patient is encountered later in the disease for the first time, one is confronted with a severe aortic stenosis with left ventricular dysfunction and possible associated valve lesions as mitral regurgitation. The impact of aortic valve replacement in these patients is unsure, the peri-operative risk seems to be very high but after surviving this phase, in the first 2 years no new mortality is added [2, 3, 4]. When aortic valve replacement is survived in patients with severe aortic stenosis and depressed left ventricular function, favorable changes develop in left ventricular mass and shape and the ejection fraction increases from 21% to 52%, accompanied by improvement in functional class [2].

When patients have developed symptoms of congestive heart failure in critical aortic stenosis, life expectancy, when untreated with valve replacement, is approximately 2 years[5]. Patients who respond well to aortic valve replacement in this group have a higher ejection fraction (32% vs 20%), higher systolic gradients across the aortic valve (peak 80 and mean 61 mmHg vs peak 28 and mean 22 mmHg) and a smaller valve area (0.21 vs 0.30) than patients who do not survive this procedure in a study in 14 patients [4]. An explanation for the latter can be that in those who do not respond well to surgery, a concomitant cardiomyopathy causes the depressed ventricular function rather than the increased wall stress imposed on by the stenotic valve. Distinguishing these patients from patients with a true critical aortic stenosis and afterload excess as principal cause of their left ventricular dysfunction, is crucial because only the latter will benefit from valve replacement.

It is well recognized that the severity of an aortic stenosis in patients with left ventricular dysfunction can be better expressed with calculation of the aortic valve area using the continuity equation than with ventricular-aortic gradients because the latter decrease with decrease of systolic function.

An even more reliable measure for this afterload mismatch is a calculation of the valve resistance instead of valve gradients or valve area[6]. This can be calculated using the formula: 1.33 x MPG x SEP / SV [7, 8], where MPG is the mean pressure gradient by continuous –wave Doppler, SEP is the systolic ejection period and SV is the stroke volume determined from the product of the left ventricular outflow tract area and the velocity time integral of the outflow tract flow.The constant 1.33 is a correction factor used to express valve resistance in dynes.s/cm5.

Necessity to have a true picture of the aortic valve resistance is needed in patients with left ventricular dysfunction, low transvalvular gradients and a severe aortic stenosis. This severe stenosis can be caused by a fixed stenotic valve or by a depressed systolic function, an inadequate driving force to open a moderately stenosed valve. Distinction between these 2 conditions is essential since only patients with a fixed stenosis will benefit from valve replacement. Dobutamine echocardiography can distinguish between these two conditions: when contractility can increase and the valve gradients and valve resistance increase and valve area remains unchanged, a true, critical severe aortic stenosis is diagnosed; when valve gradients and resistance stay unchanged and the valve area increases, a relative aortic stenosis is present where valve replacement is not the solution for the clinical problem of that patient. When contractility however can not increase, no distinction can be made and the possibility still exists that this patient has a severe aortic stenosis. These patients have a very poor prognosis[9].

In general, patients with severe aortic stenosis and left ventricular dysfunction, ejection fraction $\leq$ 35%, have a high operative mortality (10%-33%), but when they survive the operation they improve functionally and mortality is low [2, 3, 4].

CARDIAC ARGUMENTS:
AORTIC REGURGITATION, EVER TOO LATE TO OPERATE?

Noninvasive parameters for timing of surgery for chronic severe aortic regurgitation have been well developed, as discussed earlier. When symptoms develop, left ventricular endsystolic dimension approaches $26mm/m^2$ or 55 mm and enddiastolic diameter approaches $38mm/m^2$, ejection fraction falls below 40% or fractional shortening below 25-27%, valve replacement is recommended even in patients with minimal or no symptoms to prevent irreversible left ventricular dysfunction [10, 11,12].

In patients with depressed left ventricular function preoperatively, survival and improvement in ventricular function are strongly related to severity of symptoms, severity of left ventricular dysfunction and duration of ventricular dysfunction. If surgery occurs within 15 months after onset of ventricular dysfunction, restoration of function can be expected. This restoration occurs in the first 6-8 months after surgery [13].

In these patients with preoperative left ventricular dysfunction, the question arises if there are patients with such severe left ventricular dysfunction from aortic regurgitation in whom, despite the presence of a surgically correctable valve lesion, one should defer from operation because one expects no or minimal improvement after this high risk procedure.

Without surgery, deterioration is inevitable and with continued afterload mismatch heart failure will develop and outcome is poor. Aortic valve replacement, also in these patients, decompresses the ventricle and removes the increased afterload and improves the loading conditions for the ventricle. Despite the prospects of high operative risk[14] some patients with severe left ventricular dysfunction do quite well with surgery and are certainly better than preoperatively. A small minority do even better than anticipated going on to reasonable functional status and longevity.

There is probably no threshold of ejection fraction below which it is too late to operate.

Age, other concomitant diseases and the wishes of the patient and family should be taken into account in these high risk cases but in general valve replacement should be attempted even in patients in the lower ranges of ejection fraction.

If heart failure continues or progresses after surviving this operation, heart transplantation is an option.

CARDIAC ARGUMENTS :
MITRAL REGURGITATION, WHEN IS THE OPERATIVE RISK PROHIBITIVE?

In mitral regurgitation, the issue of timing of surgery, as discussed elsewhere in this course, is of extreme importance because the impact of mitral valve surgery on left ventricular function can be dramatic and true myocardial function can be never estimated correctly.

For the same degree of volume overload and increase in enddiastolic volume, patients with mitral regurgitation have reduced afterload compared with patients with aortic regurgitation [15]. Thus, estimation of the true level of left ventricular dysfunction is very difficult and is almost always overestimated with commonly used parameters as ejection fraction. This is illustrated by the observation that ejection fraction virtually in all patients declines after valve surgery and sometimes very strikingly in the individual patient [16, 17, 18]. Intraoperative observations described a better ejection fraction in patients undergoing valve repair compared to those undergoing valve replacement [19]. Mechanisms held responsible for this unfavorable influence on ventricular performance have been investigated in significant number of studies but remain still speculative. Most prominent collaborating factors are elimination of the low-pressure decompression of the left ventricle into the left atrium and disruption of the mitral apparatus in traditional valve replacement [19, 20].

The better clinical outcome in patients in whom valve repair is performed or in whom the posterior leaflet is preserved illustrates the importance of preservation or even improvement of left ventricular function after surgery for mitral regurgitation [21, 22].

When the patient is not a candidate for repair for anatomical or technical reasons, the operative and postoperative risks may be too high and with an ejection fraction in the range of 25-30% can be prohibitive. This risk not only refers to the peri-operative situation but also to the progressive long-term dysfunction and late mortality. This issue is further complicated when coronary artery disease is present. Revascularisation carries the potential for improvement in left ventricular function when viability is present and in these instances lower boundaries of function are accepted for surgery.

However, in patients with mitral regurgitation and severely depressed left ventricular function (ejection fraction below 30-40%), the perioperative risk is high and long-term survival poor [16] and this depressed ventricular function can be prohibitive, more so in patients in whom valve repair is unlikely to be successful and in whom no potential of improvement of ventricular function is expected through revascularisation of viable dysfunctioning myocardium.

CARDIAC ARGUMENTS :
MITRAL STENOSIS, NEVER TOO LATE TO OPERATE

The time from diagnosis of mild mitral stenosis to severe stenosis requiring intervention can be quite long and timing of follow-up studies will be tailored to the individual patient according to stenosis severity, coexisting cardiac abnormalities and changes in functional status. Of note, even with mild to moderate stenosis, increases in right ventricular diastolic area, tricuspid regurgitant severity and pulmonary pressures can be observed [23].

Surgical or balloon relief of mitral stenosis should be considered at the onset of symptoms or signs of pulmonary congestion.

Selection for the best interventional procedure is based on valve morphology and comorbididty. As discussed elsewhere, valve morphology can be scored [24] in a 16 point scale and when this score, describing leaflet mobility and thickening as well as the status of the subvalvular apparatus and calcification present, exceeds 8, balloon- valvuloplasty is associated with a suboptimal result and complications [25]. Of course it is hazardous to apply a rigid breakpoint for clinical decision making in patients with intermediate scores; echocardiographer, interventionalist and surgeon should review valve morphology together to decide for the most appropriate therapy. This holds true even more in patients where the surgical risk is high, patients with pulmonary hypertension. In these patients the mortality rate of surgery is high, in one study of 42 patients with pulmonary systolic pressures of 60 mmHg and higher this rate was 11.6%, as is the complication rate, in the same study 16%[26].

Predictors of death were acute presentation and signs of right ventricular hypertrophy on the electrocardiogram. Despite the high surgical risk, most patients had improved functional status and a survival rate in the first 5 years of 80%, in the first 10 years of 64%, which is significantly higher than the historical comparison of the survival rate of these patients treated medically [27].

In these patients with pulmonary hypertension, balloon-valvuloplasty is preferable but only if valve characteristics are predictive of good result. Also in these patients, echocardiographic score was the only factor independently predictive of success of the procedure [28].

Although surgical risk in patients with pulmonary hypertension is high, its is never a contraindication for surgery because it falls dramatically after relief of the obstruction.

NON-CARDIAC ARGUMENTS:
COMORBIDITY INFLUENCING THE DECISION TO DEFER FROM OPERATION

Well known variables other than cardiac ones, predictive of mortality in patients undergoing a valve or other cardiac operation with or without bypass grafting are age, decreased renal function, and chronic obstructive pulmonary disease. Furthermore the presence of active endocarditis, a prior cardiac operation , evidence of congestive heart failure, a recent myocardial infarction increase the surgical risk [29]. Patients who are at the time of operation in functional class IV are imposed on a 2.9 times greater risk of dying than those in class III. Patients in need of an emergent surgical procedure have a 4.4 times higher risk of dying versus an elective procedure [29, 30].

The influence of age on mortality is associated with the higher incidence of comorbidity in the elderly. Nevertheless, we are encountered more often with patients over 80 years of age with indications for cardiac surgery and a remarkable pile of evidence is gathered in this population and shows acceptable mortality rates, ranging from 8% to 20% [31, 32, 33, 34], and striking functional improvement [30, 35, 36].

Acute renal failure is worth mentioning in this respect because it is independently associated with early mortality after cardiac surgery, even after adjustment for comorbidity and postoperative complications [37]. When acute renal failure is present, this is a comorbidity which makes the operative risk extremely high.

Comorbidity factors as we know them nowadays all form relative contraindications for cardiac surgery, they add to the weighted cardiac risk of surgery which should be held against the possible benefit concerning prognosis and functional status after operation.

The weighed considerations should lead to a team decision of cardiac surgeons, cardiologists and intensive care specialists, especially when the critically ill patient is discussed, whether operation is the best therapeutical option for this patient.

REFERENCES

1. Pellika PA, Nishimura RA, Bailey KR, Tajik AJ: The natural history of adults with asymptomatic, hemodynamically significant aortic stenosis. J Am Coll Cardiol 1990;15:1012-1017

2. Pela G, La Canna G, Metra M, Ceconi C, Centurini PB, Alfieri O, Visioli O: Long-term changes in left ventricular mass, chamber size and function after valve replacement in patients with severe aortic stenosis and depressed ejection fraction. Cardiology 1997;88:315-322

3. Brogan WC, Grayburn PA, Lange RA, Hillis LD. Prognosis after valve replacement in patients with severe aortic stenosis and a low transvalvular pressure gradient. J Am Coll Cardiol 1993;21:1657-1660

4. Carabello BA, Green LH, Grossman W, Cohn LH, Koster JK, Collins JJ: Hemodynamic determinants of prognosis of aortic valve replacement in critical aortic stenosis and advanced congestive heart failure. Circulation 1980;62:42-48

5. Ross J jr, Braunwald E: Aortic stenosis. Circulation 1968;38[suppl V]:68

6. Cannon JD, Zile MR, Crawford FA, Carabello BA: Aoric valve resistance as an adjunct to the Gorlin formula in assessing the severity of aortic stenosis in symptomatic patients. J Am Coll Cardiol 1992;20:1517-1523

7. Ford LE, Feldman T, Chiu YC, Carroll JD: Hemodynamic resistance as a measure of functional impairment in aortic stenosis. Circ Res 1990;66:1-7

8. Ford LE, Feldman T, Carroll JD: Valve resistance. Circulation 1993;89:893-895

9. DeFilippi CR, Willett DL, Brickner E, Appleton CR, Yancy CW, Eichhorn EJ, Grayburn PA: Usefulness of dobutamine echocardiography in distinguishing severe from nonsevere valvular aortic stenosis in patients with depressed left ventricular function and low transvalvular gradients.Am J Cardiol 1995;75:191-194

10. Ross J jr: Afterload mismatch in aortic and mitral valve disease: implications for surgical therapy. J Am Coll Cardiol 1985;5:811-826

11. Bonow RO, Rosing DR, Kent KM, Epstein SE; Timing of operation for chronic aortic regurgitation. Am J Cardiol 1982;50(2):325

12. Henry WL, Bonow RO, Borer JS, et al: Observations on the optimum time for operative intervention for aortic regurgitation: I. Evaluation of the results of aortic valve replacement in symptomatic patients. Circulation 1980; 61(3):471

13. Bonow RO, Dodd JT, Maron BJ, et al: Long-term serial changes in left ventricular function and reversal of ventricular dilatation after valve replacement forchronic aortic regurgitation. Circulation 1991;78:1108-1120

14. Bonow RO, Picone AL, McIntosh CL, et al: Survival and functional results after valve replacement for aortic regurgitation from 1976-1983: Impact of preoperative left ventricular function. Circulation 1985;72:1244-1256

15. Wisenbaugh T, Spann JF, Carabello BA: Differences in myocardial performance and load betwee patients with similar amounts of chronic aortic versus chronic mitral regurgitation. J Am Coll Cardiol 1984;3:916-923

16. Phillips HR, Levine FH, Carter JE et al: Mitral valve replacement for isolated mitral regurgitation: Analysis of clinical course and late postoperative left ventricular ejection fraction. Am J Cardiol 1981;48:647-654

17. Gaasch WH, Zile MR: Left ventricular function after surgical correction of chronic mitral regurgitation. Eur Heart J 12(suppl B):48-51

18. Rozich JD, Carabello BA, Usher BW , et al: Mitral valve replacement with and without chordal preservation in patients with chronic mitral regurgitation: Mechanisms for differences in postoperative ejection performace. Circulation 1992;86:1718-1726

19. Goldman ME, Mora F, Guarino T, et al: Mitral valvuloplasty is superior to valve replacement for preservation of left ventricular function: An intraoperative two-dimensional echocardiographic study. J Am Coll Cardiol 1987;10:568-575

20. David TE, Uden DE, Strauss HD: The importance of the mitral apparatus in left ventricular function after correction of mitral regurgitation. Circulation 1983;68(suppl II): II76-II82

21. Yacoub M, Halim M, Radley-Smith R, et al: Surgical treatment of mitral regurgitation caused by floppy valves: Repair versus replacement. Circulation 1981;64(suppl II): II210-II216

22. Kaul TK, Ramsdale DR, Meek D, et al: Mitral valve replacement in patients with severe mitral regurgitation and impaired left ventricular function. Int J Cardiol 1992;35:169-179

23. Sagie A, Freitas N, Pasial LR, et al: Doppler echocardiographic assessment of long-term progression of mitral stenosis in 103 patients: valve area and right heart disease. J Am Coll Cardiol 1996;28:472-479

24. Wilkins GR, Weyman AE, Abascal VM, Block PC, Palacios IF: Percutaneous balloon dilatation of the mitral valve: an analysis of echocardiographic variables related to outcome and the mechanism of dilatation. Br Heart J 1988;60:299-308

25. Abascal VM, Wilkins GT, O'Shea JP, et al: Prediction of successful outcome of 130 patients undergoing percutaneous balloon mitral valvulotomy. Circulation 1990;82:448-456

26. Vincens JJ, Temizer D, Post JR, Edmunds LH, Herrmann HC: Long-term outcome of cardiac surgery in patients with mitral stenosis and severe pulmonary hypertension. Circulation 1995;92[suppl II]: II137-II142

27. Roy SB, Gopinath N: Mitral stenosis. Circulation 1968;38[1, suppl V]:68

28. Lefèvre T, Bonan R, Serra A, et al: Percutaneous mitral valvuloplasty in surgical high risk patients. J Am Coll Cardiol 1991;17:348-354

29. Grover FL, Hammermeister KE, Burchfiel C, and cardiac surgeons of the department of veterans affairs: Initial report of the veterans administration preoperative risk assessment study for cardiac surgery. Ann Thorac Surg 1990;50:12-28

30. Deiwick M, Tandler R, Möllhoff Th, et al: Heart surgery in patients aged eighty years and above: determinants of morbidity and mortality. Thorac Cardiovasc Surgeon 1997;45:119-126

31. Freeman WK, Schaff HV, Bri PCO, Orszulak TA, Naessens JM, Tajik AJ: Cardiac surgery in the octogenerians: Perioperative outcome and clinical follow-up. J Am Coll Cardiol 1991;18:29-35

32. Kleikamp G, Minami K, Breymann T, et al: Aortic valve replacement in octogenerians. J Heart Valve Dis 1992;1: 196-200

33. Klima U, Wimmer Geinecker G, Mair R, et al: The octogenerians- a new challenge in cardiac surgery?. Thorac Cardiovasc Surgeon 1994;42:212-217

34. Laskar M, Ghossein Y, Cornu E, Serhal C, Bertin F: Cardiac surgery in octogenerians. Is it worth it? Cardiovasc Surg 1994;2:29-30

35. Kumar P, Zehr KJ, Chang A, Baumgratner DE: Quality of life in ovtogenerians after open heart surgery. Chest 1995;108:919-926

36. Jaeger AA, Hlatky MA, Paul SM, Gortner SR: Functional capacity after cardiac surgery in elderly patients. J Am Coll Cardiol 1994;24:1040108

37. Chertow GM, Levy EM, Hammermeister KE, Grover F, Daley J: Independent association between renal failure and mortality following cardiac surgery. Am J Med 1998;104:343-348.

Section V / Chapter 2

PROSTHETIC VALVE DYSFUNCTION

**Dr. B.J.M. DELEMARRE, Dr. G.L. VAN RIJK – ZWIKKER,
Prof.Dr. R.A.E. DION**

INTRODUCTION

Prosthetic valve dysfunction is often divided into structural and non-structural valve dysfunction. However, a new condition, prosthetic valve related heart dysfunction, has been recognized, and this is attributable to the influence of the prosthesis on left ventricular function. This may ultimately also result in terminal right ventricular dysfunction. In addition, the effects of oral anticoagulant therapy instituted in patients using mechanical valve devices should to be considered. Heart dysfunction related to insertion of normally functioning prosthetic valve(s) will more frequent be encountered by cardiologists than dysfunction of the prosthetic device itself. Hence, complete discussion of valve prosthesis dysfunction needs to consider both aspects of 'prosthetic' valve dysfunction in both the mitral and aortic position, and in mechanical as well as tissue valve prostheses.

Generally, the surgeon determines whether a valve can or cannot be repaired, and which type of valve implant should be used. There are no general rules existing to indicate which type of artificial valve should be used in which kind of disease. Each type has its own advantages and disadvantages.

PROSTHESIS RELATED DYSFUNCTION, ORIENTATION

Insertion of an artificial valve in the mitral orifice implies the insertion of a rigid ring in the mitral valve annulus which will interfere with left ventricular function [1]. This will be unavoidable as long as non stented tissue valves are not routinely implanted. In the case of mechanical valve insertion in the mitral orifice, free movement of the occluder dictates the orientation of the prosthesis [2].

At present two types of mechanical valve prostheses are used: the disc valve and the bileaflet valve. The occluder(s) of both types change the inflow direction of the bloodstream into the left ventricle. The occluder of the disc valve prosthesis deflects the flow into the direction of the greater orifice. In the bileaflet prosthesis, the round orifice is divided into two equal parts by the hinge line. Flow through the valve results in two symmetrical jets [3].

In the disc valve prosthesis, orientation of the greater orifice towards the septum results in an inflow stream directed towards the septum. *(FIG 1A)* This bloodstream continues on its way during diastole, along the lateral wall towards the base of the heart. On its way to the outflow tract, it will collide with blood entering the left ventricle. Concomitant with this flow pattern, one may often observe an abnormal motion of the interventricular septum, apparently induced by the early diastolic bloodstream directed towards the septum. If the disc valve is oriented with the greater orifice towards the lateral wall, the inflow is directed towards the lateral wall. In this orientation, the diastolic bloodstream away from the apex can enter unimpeded the outflow tract. *(FIG 1B)* In the long-term, this proved to be more advantageous in as much as there were lower gradients across the valve, lower wedge pressures and less occurrence of atrial fibrillation [4,5].

A bileaflet mechanical valve prosthesis can be implanted either with the hinge line parallel with the interventricular septum (anatomical orientation) or with the hinge line perpendicular to the septum (anti-anatomical orientation). In the case of a bileaflet valve prosthesis, the two major inflow jets determine the flow pattern. As described by our group, the left ventricular spatial flow pattern will change dramatically [6]. Although it is generally accepted that the blood flow pattern through a bileaflet valve prosthesis is symmetrical, this does not mean that changing the orientation of this valve always results in an identical spatial flow pattern. The location of an outflow tract adjacent to an inflow tract, results in an asymmetrical left ventricular inflow tract, if the prosthesis is orientated with the hinge line parallel with the septum, the anatomical orientation. The septal directed orifice leads to a wider inflow tract, consisting of half an inflow path together with the entire outflow tract. The other major orifice is oriented towards half the inflow path formed by the lateral wall. Hence, the inflow jet through this orifice will maintain a higher velocity than the inflow jet through the septal oriented orifice. These two flow streams merge at the apical part of the septum. The septally oriented inflow stream prevents the diastolic blood flow (which is away from the apex) from entering the outflow tract, and thus the blood flow is diverted towards the valve prosthesis, leading to its asymmetrical and premature closure. *(FIG 2, panel A+B)* Both in patients in whom the greater orifice of a disc valve is oriented towards the septum, and in patients with an anatomically oriented bileaflet valve, similar abnormal septal motion is observed. The septum moves with an early diastolic motion towards the right ventricular cavity, leading to an abnormally weaving movement.

In contrast, if a bileaflet valve is oriented with the hinge line perpendicular to the septum (the anti-anatomical orientation), the left ventricle is divided into two symmetrical parts consisting of half the inflow tract and half the outflow tract. Inflow therefore, consists of two symmetrical inflow streams: one along the anterior wall and one along the posterior wall. These streams will unite at the apex, causing a diastolic apical bloodstream away from the apex which moves between the two inflow jets towards the base. This results in a complex three layered flow pattern during diastole, in which the middle layer can enter the outflow tract unimpeded.

(FIG 3, panel A+B) Occluder closure is symmetrical, and as there is no preferential blood flow directed towards the septum, abnormal septal motion is seldom observed in this orientation. These flow patterns may easily be interpreted using color Doppler echocardiography. In order to overcome the problem of a low frame rate, it is

advisable to make long recordings, as the short-lasting periods in spatial flow investigation can easily be missed.

In a group of 56 patients with a non-dilated left ventricle we have encountered abnormal septal motion more frequently in patients with the anatomical orientation of the prosthesis [15/31], than in patient with the anti-anatomical orientation [4/25]. Thus, the latter orientation may be preferable.

Bio-prostheses have the advantage of a central inflow and hence the normal diastolic flow pattern within the left ventricle. This only occurs if the valve is correctly oriented with the ostium towards the apex. However, in the case of an enlarged left atrium or annular dilatation, insertion of such a prosthesis may result in an off-axis orientation, with abnormal deviation of the inflow towards the septum. *(FIG 4, panel A+B)* This may cause the same flow pattern as observed in patients with a disc valve prosthesis in the mitral valve annulus (oriented with the greater orifice towards the septum), resulting in the same deleterious effects. The implantation direction of a bio-prosthesis can easily be recognized, using two-dimensional echocardiography. (Note that in patients with a normal apically directed bio-prosthesis, deviation of the inflow away from the apex may be an early indication of valve deterioration.)

PROSTHESIS RELATED DYSFUNCTION, SUBVALVULAR APPARATUS

Although several papers exist proving that the subvalvular apparatus has to be saved to maintain left ventricular function, still randomized papers are published concerning this subject [7-12]. However, it is not always possible to prevent the necessity for resection of the subvalvular apparatus because of thickening and or retraction of the chords. If the basal chords are resected, the continuation between the cardiac base and apex is destroyed. In particular, the 'aortic root-left ventricular lateral wall' axis will be lost once the basal chords originating from the antero-lateral papillary muscle leading to the anterior leaflet are severed. This will result in a spherical shape of the left ventricle instead of an oval shape. The oval shape is preferable for ejection of blood out of the left ventricle. Hence, preservation results in smaller left ventricular volume and higher ejection fraction [7,8]. The effect of resecting the chords will partically in the dilated left ventricle, be deleterious as demonstrated by Hansen. In their canine study a diminished left ventricular peak pressure, dp/dt and higher left ventricular end diastolic pressure was described [11].

To date no general experience exists concerning the insertion and sizing of artificial chords in patients in whom the subvalvular apparatus needs excision. However, with increasing experience the results will improve [13].

In the aortic valve position, there is also a preferential implantation orientation for mechanical disc valve prosthesis: the greater orifice should be oriented towards the right posterior aortic wall. This orientation seems more important with the smaller sized prostheses [14]. Using this orientation, flow through the valve prosthesis complied most with physiological conditions [15]. The different orientations in the aortic root have influence on turbulence downstream from the valve as far as into the aortic arch [16]. The bileaflet prosthesis seems on one hand less dependent of orientation, but on the other hand it has less favorable dynamics than the disc prosthesis [15.] This preferential orientation is the result of the deviation of the blood stream by the occluder and therefore the situation does not apply in tissue valves.

What is important for the cardiologist?
Although it is fairly easy for the cardiologist to evaluate the above mentioned conditions, nothing can be changed once the operation is completed and the patient is evaluated on the outpatient ward. The surgeon should therefore be informed prior to the operation, of the nature and mechanism of the disease, of what might be expected at the time of operation, and of which chords can or cannot be saved. In addition, left and right ventricular function, pulmonary artery pressure and (in the case of a reoperation), the presence or absence of paravalvular leakage should be mentioned. Depending all these data, advise may be given on the type of prosthesis to be used and the orientation of the valve. During or immediately after the operation, the valve orientation can be investigated and adjustments made easily and with less additional risk for the patient.

What is the relevance for the patient?
Before the operation, the cardiologist should discuss with the patient the feasibility of valve repair or replacement, the advantages and disadvantages of mechanical versus tissue valve prosthesis. He should explain to the patient what he or she might expect from the operation regarding life expectancy and exercise tolerance, so that a personal decision can be made. This type of question relates to the above mentioned conditions. Indeed, the patient should, if asked, be informed of his or her prognosis. After the operation he or she can be informed that everything is, to the best of our knowledge, satisfactory, and that a normal lifestyle can be resumed or that restrictions remain.
In this way, we can at least gain some insight into the relationship between underlying pathology and best suited valve prosthesis for a particular patient (i.e. the influence of valve prosthesis design on left and right ventricular function.) Thus we may gather information on the relation between underlying valve pathology and prognosis after valve prosthesis implantation. The cardiologist therefore has to consider and evaluate the above mentioned aspects before and during the operation, since at the time of intervention decisions can be made to optimize these aspects for the particular patient. After the operation the situation is definitive.

DYSFUNCTION OF THE VALVE PROSTHESIS, STRUCTURAL

A complication present from the moment of operation but which is a seldom met form of prosthetic dysfunction, is patient-valve prosthesis mismatch. It might appear in children with a valve prosthesis in puberty and in older patients with degenerative aortic valve stenosis and a hypoplastic aortic root. After mitral valve replacement, a normal pressure half time in combination with high gradients and PAP-pressure, without abnormal mitral regurgitation may be indicative of this diagnosis. After aortic valve replacement, high gradients with a, for the diameter of the valve, normal functional area sometimes account for this diagnosis. The introduction of non-stented valve prostheses is the main reason for this diagnosis rarely being encountered [17].

The more usual forms of prosthesis dysfunction can be divided into structural and non-structural dysfunction. In structural valve dysfunction it is the prosthesis itself that malfunctions due to mechanical failure. This form of valve dysfunction is often related to type and size. In contrast, in non-structural valve dysfunction, an in principal curable disease, e.g. thrombus formation, endocarditis etc., causes the valve prosthesis to malfunction and hence all patients carry the same risk.

Mechanical valve prosthesis dysfunction can be caused by fracture of the static material, leading to occluder dislodgement. Disc embolisation is well known in the Björk-Shiley prosthesis due to fracture of the welded outlet strut [18]. Less well known is the fact that cavitation, induced by the high motion velocity of the valve leaflets, may damage the occluder and may finally lead to fracture and embolisation of the occluder [19,20]. One should suspect this condition if a healthy patient deteriorates acutely and prosthesis sounds are absent. Immediate intervention with valve replacement is the only chance for patient survival.

Bio-prostheses dysfunction due to degeneration of the valve biomaterial induced by the fixation process or due to stent fracture. Tissue valves degenerate over time by calcification, tearing or perforation. Calcification has inversely been related with the age of the recipient at the moment of implantation and with high pressure tissue fixation with gluteraldehyde [21]. Low pressure fixed valves appear to be more durable [22]. In addition, there have been bio-prosthesis models designed to optimize the flow profile through the valve and to diminish the gradient across the valve. In particular some Pericardial valves turned out to be prone to valve deterioration due to accelerated tissue tearing [23,24]. Using the older type of echo-equipment, visualization of the valve tissue within the stent may be an indication for tissue calcification.

Using the newer type of equipment, cusp motion may easily be recorded. Deviation of the flow direction over time through the valve is a more sophisticated sign of bio-prosthesis degeneration. In addition, tissue tearing or perforation causes newly developed valve regurgitation.

Using two dimensional Doppler echocardiography, prevalvular flow acceleration may indicate prosthetic valve regurgitation[25]. Conventional Doppler echocardiography may also be used in order to detect this. Peak velocity of mitral inflow (>1.9 m/s), mean gradient (>5mmHg) and the ratio of the time velocity integral of the mitral inflow to the time velocity integral in the left ventricular outflow tract (>2.5) have been described as indicators of prosthetic valve regurgitation[26].

As stentless bioprostheses do not have a solid structure, incorrect sizing may lead to difficulties. In pigs we have demonstrated that a too small valve within the aortic root leads to stretching of the valve cusps, leading to mal coaptation; on the other hand oversizing may lead to plication and folding of the valve cusps. This results in early degeneration of the valve cusps[27]. Both conditions cause aortic valve incompetence.

There are few reports on the long-term function of stentless valves. However, reports on valvular dysfunction of freehand grafts, describe proximal suture line dehiscence. This is a complication which, if going unnoticed, may lead to death of the patient as the valve turns inside out [28].

DYSFUNCTION OF THE VALVE PROSTHESIS, NON STRUCTURAL

A form of non-structural valve dysfunction, sometimes present from the moment of operation, is valve incompetence due to paravalvular leakage. Paravalvular leakage is related to annular calcification, endocarditis at the moment of operation and re-operation [29]. Paravalvular defects in the mitral position have a predilection for the postero commisural area [30]. Only on patients with left ventricular failure caused by the incompetent valve, or who needed multiple blood transfusions due to hemolysis caused by the regurgitant jet, was re-operation performed. A more aggressive approach is currently advised [29]. New developments such as silver coating of the suture ring of the St Jude Medical prosthesis, in order to protect the patient against early bacterial endocarditis, have proved unhelpful. The silver coating may have prevented tissue overgrowth of the ring and hence facilitated paravalvular leakage [31,32]. Newly acquired paravalvular leakage may be caused, early post-operatively, by valve dehiscence due to stitch rupture. At any time it may be caused by endocarditis, which is a very serious disease with a high mortality rate even in the area of surgical treatment [33].

Absence of occluder motion can occur early after operation by entrapment of stitches by the prosthesis, or by interference with native valve remnants, myocardium or vessel wall [2,34]. In particular, entrapment of a stitch by a mitral valve prosthesis causes a serious condition since the closing force exceeds many times the opening force i.e. the diastolic pressure difference between left atrium and the left ventricle. In the case of malfunction of the prosthesis by interference with surrounding structures, the only treatment is immediate reoperation.

Obstruction of blood flow through the valve prosthesis resulting from tissue overgrowth or thrombus formation on the valve causes abnormal or absence of occluder motion [35]. Pannus formation can be suspected if the gradients across the valve prosthesis increases, pulmonic pressure gradually increases and cardiac output decreases. Direct visualization using transesophageal echocardiography is not easy, as the metal valve ring induces strong echo reflections and hence hampers image formation. After the diagnosis has been made, the treatment consists of reoperation. Thrombus formation on a mechanical valve prosthesis can be suspected in patients with inadequate anticoagulation. It can be detected by abnormal occluder motion using X-ray examination, by increasing gradients across the valve prosthesis *(FIG 5)* and by an approximation of peak and mean gradient *(FIG 6)*. Thrombus formation can often be visualized by transesophageal echocardiography [36] *(FIG 7)*. Initial therapy may consist of thrombolysis with streptokinase or tPA, which may prove to be a life saving procedure [37]. This treatment usually forms a bridge to operation, as surgical cleaning of the valve or valve replacement is the definitive treatment. Thrombus formation can sometimes be linked to a particular type of valve design, such as the Medtronic Parallel TM bileaflet valve [38].

Often reported as having a valve prosthesis dysfunction and always difficult to treat, is the patient with a transient ischemic attack, referred by the neurologist for exclusion of a cardiac source of emboli. In addition to the normal transthoracic echo examination with determination of gradients, valve area or pressure half time (to give an indication of whether or not valve obstruction exists) transeophageal echocardiography should be performed. In these patients one can encounter echostrands, thin fibrous thread like structures, spontaneous contrast in the left atrium and high intensity transient signals, all conditions which are associated with cardiac emboli in the literature. Unfortunately, these conditions can also be found in patients with valve prosthesis, who do not have neurological disorders [39]. The main issue is whether or not to replace the valve in these patients, since insertion of another valve prosthesis will often result in the same phenomena.

It can be deduced from the above mentioned that Doppler echocardiography plays a major role in the diagnosis of valve prosthesis dysfunction. It is mandatory to document the function of the prosthesis in the early postoperative state, in order to be able to detect changes in the function of the prosthesis. Of equal importance is the adequate archiving of the results so that they remain available in the future. In the case of a mitral valve prosthesis, early Doppler echocardiographic examination should be used to determine peak and mean gradients, pressure half time, presence or absence of paravalvular leakage and the, for the particular prosthesis, normal flow through the prosthesis. In addition, the pulmonary artery pressure should be determined at rest as well as after exercise, as patients may show an abnormal hemodynamic response on exercise [40]. All these parameters may be obtained using transthoracic echocardiography. Although the paravalvular leakage jet itself cannot be visualized by the masking effect of the prosthetic material, the flow acceleration in front of the regurgitant orifice can often be visualized and thus should be looked for. The jet can be unmasked using transesophageal echocardiography. In the case of an aortic valve prosthesis peak and mean gradient, functional aortic valve area and paravalvular leakage should be documented. In contrast to patients with a mitral valve prosthesis, the "physiological" leakage backflow particular to the valve prosthesis can often be recorded in patients with aortic valve prosthesis.

Thus, other than valve related dysfunction, dysfunction of the valve prosthesis itself is a treatable disease. Once a patient with a valve prosthesis begins to complain about a diminished exercise tolerance, one has to consider the possibility of prosthesis dysfunction; by just comparing two Doppler echocardiographic investigations the diagnosis can be made.

170

REFERENCES

1. v Rijk-Zwikker GL, Schipperheyn JJ, Huysmans HA 1989 Influence of mitral valve prosthesis or rigid mitral ring on left ventricular function. Circulation 80, 1-7.
2. Hall KV 1988 Surgical considerations for avoiding disc interference based on a ten year experience with the Medtronic Hall heart valve. J Card Surg 3, 103-108.
3. Yoganathan AP, McMillan ST, Woo RY, Sung HW In vitro evaluation of prosthetic heart valves by Doppler flow imaging. In Nanda NC ed, Textbook of color Doppler echocardiography, Lea & Febiger 1989 Philadelphia, Londen p.312-318.
4. Björk VO, Book K, Holmgren A. 1974 The Björk – Shiley mitral valve prosthesis: a comparative study with different prosthesis orientations Ann Thorac Surg 18, 379-386.
5. Pop G, Sutherland GR, Roelandt J, Vletter W, Bos E. 1989 What is the ideal orientation of a mitral disc prosthesis? An in vivo haemodynamic study based on color flow imaging and continuous Wave Doppler. European H J 10, 346-353.
6. v Rijk-Zwikker GL, Delemarre BJ, Huysmans HA. 1996 The orientation of the bileaflet CarboMedics valve in the mitral position determines left ventricular spatial flow patterns. Eur J Cardio-thorac Surg 10, 513-520.
7. David TE, Burns RJ, Bacchus CM, Druck MN. 1984 Mitral valve replacement for mitral regurgitation with and without preservation of chordae tendineae. J Thorac Cardiovasc Surg 88, 718-725.
8. Rozich JD, Carabello Ba, Usher BW, Kratz JM, Bell AE, Zile MR. 1992 Mitral valve replacement with and without chordal preservation in patients with chronic mitral regurgitation. Mechanisms for differences in postoperative ejection performance. Circulation 86, 1718-1726.
9. David TE, Armstrong S, Zhao Sun BA. 1995 Left ventricular function after mitral valve surgery. J Heart Valve Dis 4, S175- S180.
10. Lee EM, Shapiro LM, Wells FC. 1996 Importance of subvalvular preservation and early operation in mitral valve surgery. Circulation 94, 2117-2123.
11. Hansen DE, Cahill PD, DeCampli WM, Harrison DC, Derby GC, Mitchell RS, Miller DG. 1986 Valvular-ventricular interaction: importance of the mitral apparatus in canine left ventricle systolic performance. Circulation 73, 1310-1320.
12. Popovic Z, BaracI, Jovic M, Panic G, Miric M, Bojic M. 1999 Ventricular performance following valve replacement for chronic mitral regurgitation: importance of chordal preservation. J Cardiovasc Surg 40, 183-190.
13. El Khoury G, Noirhomme P, Verhelst R, Rubay J, Dion R 2000 Surgical repair of the prolapsing anterior leaflet in degenerative mitral valve disease. J Heart Valve Dis 9;75-81.
14. Laas J, Kleine P, Hasenkam MJ, Nygaard H 1999 Orientation of tilting disc and bileaflet aortic valve substitutes for optimal hemodynamics. Ann Thorac Surg 68, 1096-1099.
15. Kleine P, Perthel M, Nygaard H, Hansen SB, Paulsen PK, Riis C, Laas J 1998 Medtronic Hall versus St. Jude Medical mechanical aortic valve: Downstream turbulence with respect to rotation in pigs. J Heart Valve Dis 7, 548-855.
16. Chandran KB, Khalighi B, Chen CJ, 1985 Experimental study of physiological pulsatile flow past valve prosthesis in a model of human aorta – II Tilting disc valves and effect of orientation J Biomech 18, 773-780.
17. Baur LHB, Yin XY, Houdas Y, Peels CH, Braun J, Kappetein AP, Prat A, Hazekamp MG, v Straten BHM, Ploeg A, Sieders A, Voogd PJ, Bruschke AVG, vd Wall EE, Westaby S, Huysmans HA 1999 Echocardiographic parameters of the Freestyle stentless biprosthesis in aortic position: the European experience J Am Soc Echocardiogr 12;729-735.

18. Wieting DW, Eberhardt AC, Reul H, Breznock EM, Schneck SG, Chandler JG 1999. Strut fracture mechanisms of the Bjork-Shiley convexo-concave heart valve. J Heart Valve Dis 8,206-217.

19. Klepetko W, Moritz A. 1989 Leaflet fracture in Duromedics- Edwards bileaflet valves. J Thorac Cardiovasc Surg 97;90-94.

20. Graf T, Reul H, Detlefs C, Wilmes R, Rau G. 1994 Causes and formation of cavitation in mechanical heart valves J Heart Valve Disease 3; S49-64.

21. Jamieson WR, Rosade LJ, Munro AI,Gerein AN, Burr LH, Miyagishima RT, Janusz MT, Tyers GF 1988. Carpentier-Edwards standard porcine bioprosthesis – primary tissue failure (structural valve deterioration) by age groups. Ann Thorac Surg 46;155-162.

22. Christie GW, Gross JF, Eberhardt CE 1999 Fatigue-induced changes to the biaxial mechanical properties of glutaraldehyde-fixed porcine aortic valve leaflets. Semin Thorac Cardiovasc Surg 11;S201-205.

23. Jamieson WR, Burr LH, Janusz MT, Munro AI, Hayden RI, Miyagishi RT, Ling H, Fradet GJ, Lichtenstein SV, Stewart KM 1999. Carpentier-Edwards standard and supraannular porcine bioprosthesis: comparison of technology. Ann Thorac Surg 67:10-17.

24. Naqvi TZ, Siegel RJ, Buchbinder NA, Miroshnik S, Saedi G, Trento A, Fishbein MC 1999 chocardiographic and pathologic features of explanted Hancoc and Carpentier-Edwards bioprosthetic valves in the mitral position. Am J Cardiol 84, 1422-1427.

25. Yoshida K, Yoshikawa J, Akasaka T, Nishigami K, Minagoe S 1992 Value of acceleration flow signals proximal to the leaking orifice in assessing the severity of prosthetic mitral valve regurgitation. J Am Coll Cardiol 19, 333-338

26. Olmos L, Salazar G, Barbetseas J, Qiunones MA, Zoghbi WA 1999 Usefulness of transthoracic echocardiography in detecting significant prosthetic mitral valve regurgitation. Am J Cardiol 83, 199- 205.

27. v Rijk-Zwikker GL, Delemarre BJ, Vrancken Peeters MP, Hazekamp M, Huysmans HA 1994 Observations in oversized porcine allografts in the pig. In New Horizons and Future of Heart Valve Bioprotheses. Gabbay S, Frater RWM, Eds. Silent Partners, Inc., Austin©. Chapter 18,p245-258.

28. Schoof PH, Baur LH, Kappetein AP, Hazekamp MG, van Rijk-Zwikker GL, Huysmans HA 1999. Dehiscence of the Freestyle stentless bioprosthesis. Semin Thorac Cardiovasc Surg 11;133-138.

29. Genoni M, Franzen D, Vogt P, Seifert B, Jenni R, Kunzli A, Niederhaus A, Turina M 2000 aravalvular leakage after mitral valve replacement: improved long-term survival with aggressive surgery? Eur J Cardiothorac Surg 17;14-19.

30. van Rijk-Zwikker GL, Huysmans HA 1986 The incidence and localization of para-valvular leaks in combined aortic and mitral valve replacement. In: Proceedings international workshop on the management of multivalvular heart disease. Nitterhauge S., ed Oslo, Norway p24-29.

31. Schaff H, Carrel T, Steckelberg JM, Grunkemeier GL, Holubkov R 1999. Artificial Valve Endocarditis Reduction Trial (AVERT): protocol of a multicenter randomized trial. J Heart Valve Dis 8;131-139.

32. Herold U, De Wal H, Piotrowski J, Jacob H 2000 Disruption of the silver and non-silver coated sewing cuff of a new generation bileaflet valve prosthesis during aortic valve replacement: report on four cases. Eur J Cardiothorac Surg 18;225-227.Durack DT, Lukes AS, Bright DK 1994 New criteria for the diagnosis of infective endocarditis: utilization of echocardiographic findings. Duke endocarditis service. Am J Med 96;200-209.

33. Baudet ME, Oca CC, Roques XF, Patra P, Train M, Dupon H, Rozo L, Carlier R 1985 A five and half year experience with the St Jude Medical cardiac valve prosthesis. J Thorac Cardiovasc Surg 90;137-144.

34. Rizzoli G, Guglielmi C, Toscano G, Pistorio V, Vendramin I, Bottio T, Thiene G, Casarotto D. 1999 Reoperations for acute prosthetic thrombosis and pannus: an assessment of rates, relationship and risk. European J Cardio-Thoracic Surg 16;74-80.

35. Montorsi P, De Bernardi F, Muratori M, Cavoretto D, Pepi M 2000 Role of cine-fluoroscopy, transthoracic, and transesophageal echocardiography in patients with suspected prosthetic valve thrombosis. Am J Cardiol 85, 58-64.

36. Shapira Y, Herz I, Vaturi M, Porter A, Adler Y, Birnbaum Y, Strasberg B, Sclarovsky S, Sagie A.

37. 2000 Thrombolysis is an effective and safe therapy in stuck bileaflet mitral valves in the absence of high-risk thrombi J Am Coll Cardiol 35, 1874-1880.

38. Ellis JT, Healy TM, Fontaine AA, Saxena R, Yoganathan AP 1996. Velocity measurements and flow patterns within the hinge region of a Medtronic Parallel TM bileaflet mechanical valve with clear housing J Heart Valve Dis 5:591-599.

39. Manning J 1997 Role of ttransesophageal echocardiography in the management of thromboembolic stroke Am J Cardiol 80;19D-28D.

40. Nellesen U, Inserlmann G, Ludwig J, Jahns R, Capell AJ, Eigel P 2000 Rest and exercise hemodynamics before and after valve replacement – a combined Doppler/catheter study. Clin Cardiol 23;32-38.

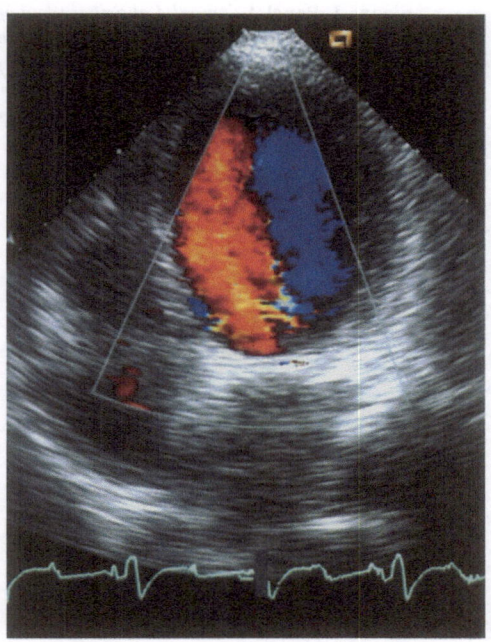

Figure 1a. *Two dimensional Doppler recording of the left ventricular spatial flow pattern caused by a disc valve prosthesis in the mitral valve ostium. The greater orifice has been oriented towards the interventricular septum. The inflow, red colour, is deviated towards the septum. The diastolic flow away from the apex (blue colour), moves along the lateral wall towards the base of the heart. Its continuous motion towards the outflow tract is blocked by the inflow stream. The resulting spatial flow pattern consists of an apical whirl rotating clockwise.*

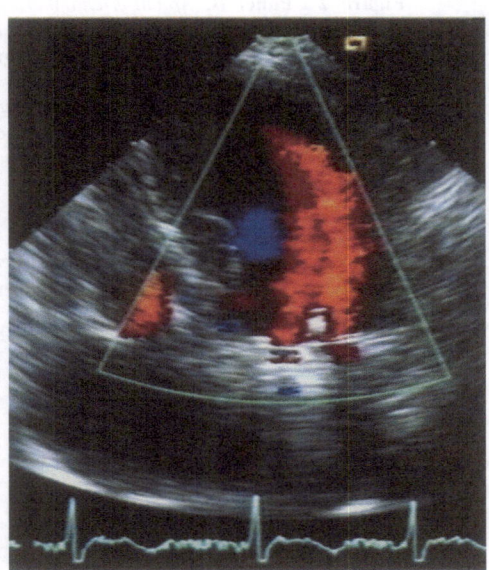

Figure 1b. *Two dimensional Doppler recording of the left ventricular spatial flow pattern caused by a disc valve prosthesis with the greater orifice oriented towards the lateral wall. The inflow (red colour) is directed towards the lateral wall. The diastolic flow away from the apex along the interventricular septum (blue colour) may enter the left ventricular outflow tract unimpeded. The spatial flow pattern is characterised by an apical whirl, rotating counter clockwise.*

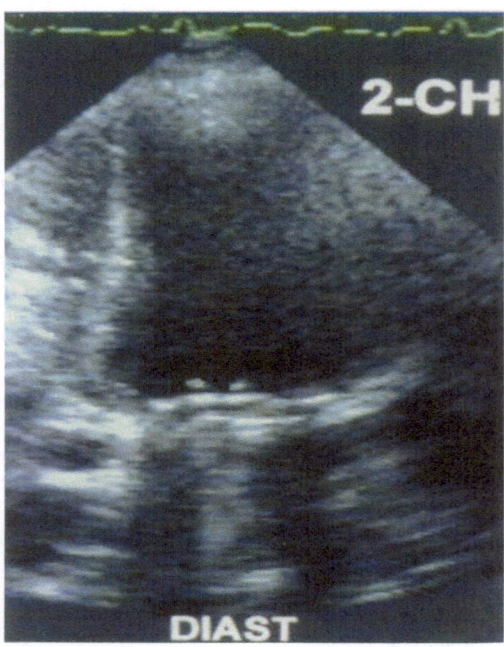

Figure 2 Panel A. *Apical 4 chamber view of a bileaflet valve prosthesis in the mitral orifice, implanted in the anatomical orientation (hinge line parallel with the interventricular septum). In the apical 4 chamber view during diastole two leaflets can separately be discerned.*

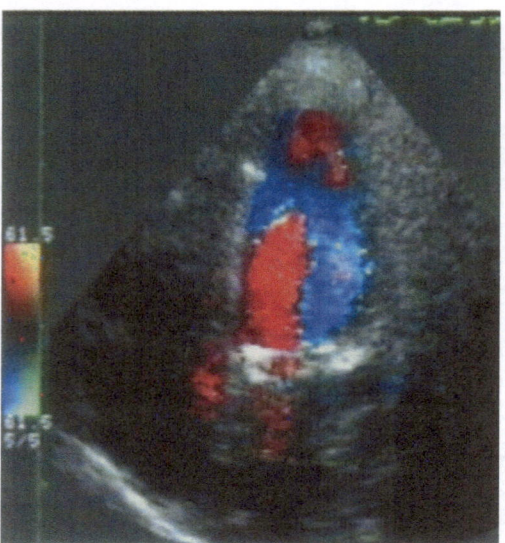

Figure 2 Panel B. *Apical 4-chamber, two dimensional Doppler recording of the left ventricular spatial flow pattern induced by a bileaflet valve prosthesis inserted in the anatomical orientation. The left ventricular spatial flow pattern is characterised by one inflow jet directed towards the interventricular septum and one inflow jet directed towards the lateral wall. Both flow streams merge at the apex. The diastolic blood flow away from the apex between the two inflow jets is directed towards the prosthesis and is prevented from entering the left ventricular outflow tract*

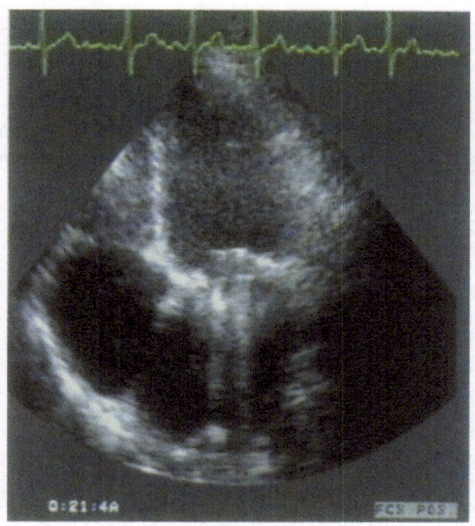

Figure 3 Panel A. *Apical 2 chamber view of a bileaflet valve prosthesis in the mitral orifice, implanted in the anti-anatomical orientation (hinge line perpendicular to the interventricular septum). In the 2 chamber view during diastole the two leaflets can separately be discerned.*

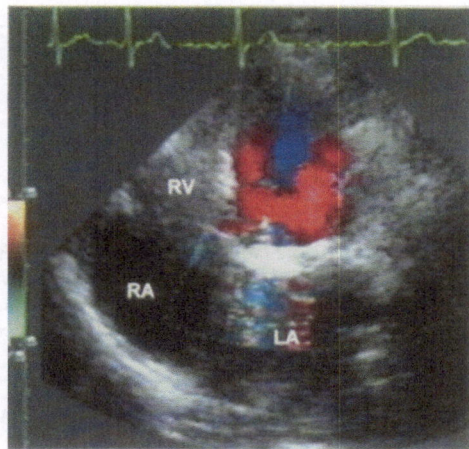

Figure 3 Panel B. *Apical 4-chamber, two dimensional Doppler recording of the left ventricular spatial flow pattern caused by a bileaflet valve prosthesis inserted in the anti-anatomical orientation. In the vicinity of the valve prosthesis, a red flow stream is recorded, indicating blood motion towards the transducer. Mid ventricular, a blue colour is recorded, indicating blood motion away from the transducer. In the apex again a red colour is recorded, indicating blood motion in the direction of the transducer. The left ventricular spatial flow pattern is characterised by three layers of blood motion: two layers of blood moving towards the apex (one along the anterior wall and one along the posterior wall) with one layer of blood moving towards the cardiac base in between. This bloodstream may enter the outflow tract unimpeded. The Doppler recording results from a scanplane that cuts trough the three separate layers.*

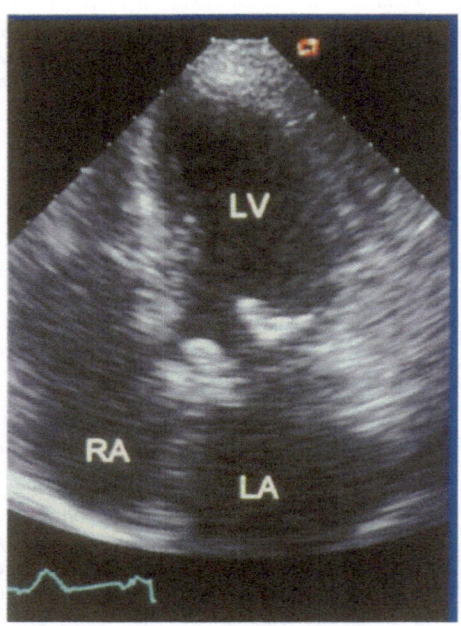

Figure 4A. *Apical 4-chamber view of a bioprosthesis oriented towards the interventricular septum instead of towards the apex.*

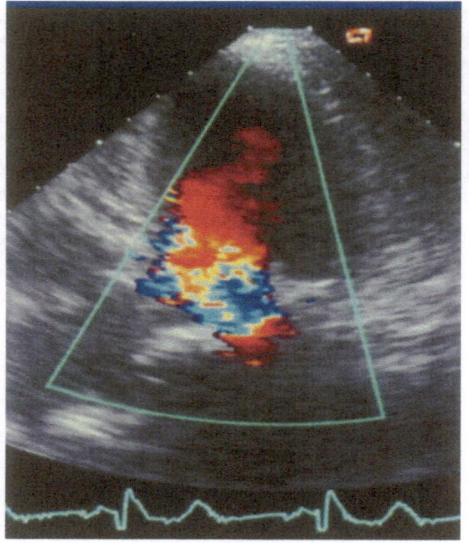

Figure 4B. *The blood stream through the valve is deviated towards the interventricular septum and hence a spatial flow pattern results that can be characterised by a clockwise rotating apical whirl.*
(compare Fig 1a)

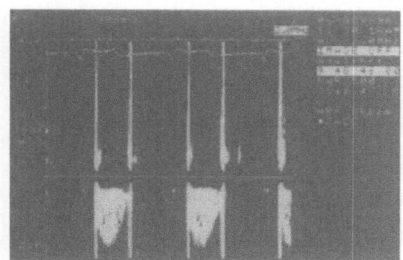

Panel (6-11-'96) recording early after aortic valve replacement for congenital aortic stenosis (peak gradient 16 mmHg). The artefacts caused by opening and
closing of the valve, encompass the flow velocity recording (arrow A) Closure backflow is not recorded (arrow B).

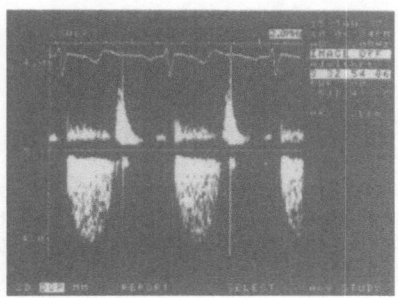

Panel (15-1-'97). Doppler recording after this patient admitted himself with complaints of dizziness. Oral anticoagulant therapy was stopped after a visit to the dentist. The peak gradient had increased to 96 mmHg. A clear delay existed between end systole (stop blood motion) and closure of the valve prosthesis (arrow A). A closure backflow could obviously be recorded (arrow B).

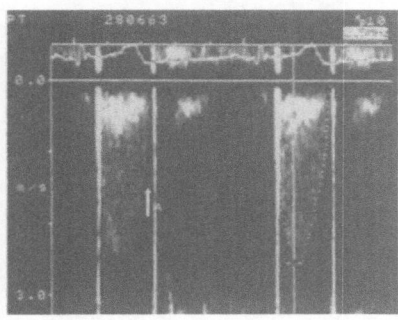

Panel 26-2-'97. After operation and cleaning of the valve prosthesis, a peak gradient of 25 mmHg was recorded. Opening and closing artefacts encompass the flow velocity recording again
(arrow A) and a closure backflow could no longer be recorded.

Figure 5. *Continuous Wave Doppler recordings of blood flow through a Medtronic Hall aortic valve prosthesis*

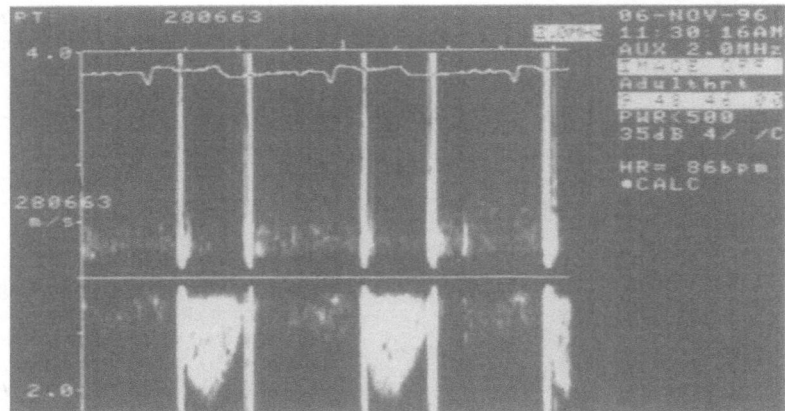

Figure 6. *Transesophageal continuous wave Doppler recording of blood flow across a mitral disc valve prosthesis obstructed by thrombus formation. The mean gradient approaches the peak gradient. This caused by a decreased cardiac output, in combination with a pressure difference between left atrium and left ventricle that remains almost the same during diastole.*

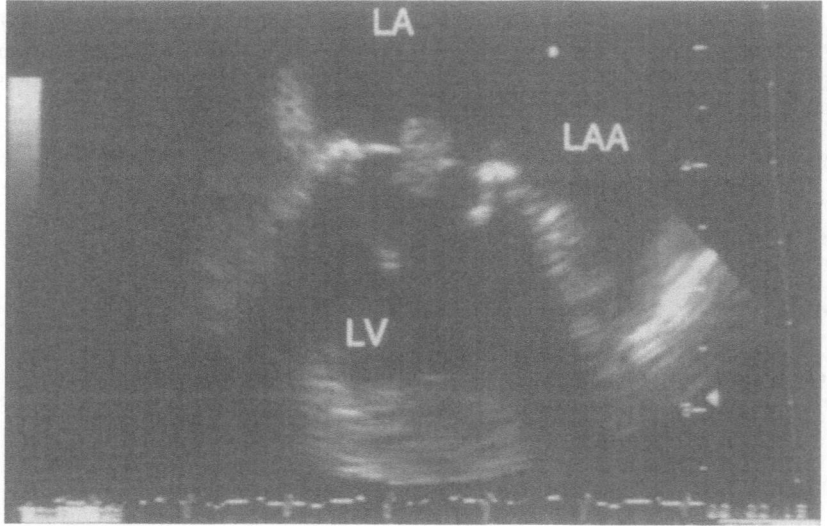

Figure 7. *Transesophageal echocardiographic recording of a thrombus in a bio prosthesis*

Section V / Chapter 3

VALVULAR PATHOLOGY IN PREGNANCY

Dr. K. KONINGS, Dr. F.J.M.E. ROUMEN, Dr. L.H. B. BAUR

INTRODUCTION

Valvular pathology and pregnancy can greatly influence each other's symptoms. Pregnancy increases the demands of the maternal cardiovascular system and thereby may aggravate symptoms due to valve disease. This can cause great risk to the health of the mother. On the other hand, valvular disease may limit the mother's ability to fulfill the needs of the growing fetus. This may lead to fetal morbidity and mortality. Potential negative effects on the fetus may also restrict therapeutic options. Therefore, early and adequate risk stratification of pregnant women with valvular pathology is essential.

Clinical diagnosis of valvular dysfunction in pregnancy may be confusing, since the symptoms of normal pregnancy can imitate those of valvular pathology. Complaints of fatigue, dyspnea, orthopnea, malleolar edema and faintness are common. Physical examination often reveals a strong abrupt pulse (as found in aortic insufficiency), jugular venous distention and a systolic flow murmur. The ECG may show aspecific changes in axis and STT-segments. Chest X-ray is not recommended because of the negative effects on the fetus. The confusion may be even greater if one considers that the cardiovascular adaptation to pregnancy occasionally reveals a previously unnoticed valvular abnormality. Therefore, caution is warranted and echocardiography is recommended in cases of doubt. Echo-Doppler measurements are the diagnostic examination of choice, since they assure the most valuable information on the severity of valvular lesions, measure left and right ventricular function and atrial size[1]. Caution is necessary, because valvular lesions can be underestimated during pregnancy[1].

Pregnant women with previously diagnosed valvular pathology should be under close supervision of an obstetrician and cardiologist. Echocardiography is the technique of choice for diagnosis and determination of the severity of the disease. Development of symptoms is an indication for sequential echocardiographic examination. Provisions for delivery with hemodynamic monitoring should be available, if required. In some cases, obstetric or cardiac intervention is unavoidable. This article is guided by an excellent overview on valvular heart disease in pregnancy by Teerlink and Foster[2], and reviews several other recent publications,[3-8] together with some observations on aortic dissection during pregnancy.[9-12]

PREGNANCY AND VALVE PATHOLOGY; PHYSIOLOGICAL ADAPTATION

During pregnancy the cardiovascular system of the mother adapts in order to fulfill the needs of the growing fetus. A scala of neurohumoral responses occur to achieve this adaptation[2]. High estrogen levels and an increased sympathetic nervous tone stimulate the renin-angiotensin-aldosterone system, cause water and salt retention, and thus increase plasma volume and increase heart rate and ventricular stroke volume already starting at the fifth wek of pregnancy with a maximum around 24 to 28 weeks of pregnancy. The pregnant state also stimulates erythropoesis, but to a lesser degree than plasma volume, developing a physiologic anemia. The low resistance of the total (including the placental) circulation decreases systemic vascular resistance. Overall, these changes result in a larger total blood volume, a physiologic left ventricular hypertrophy[5] and a 30-50% rise in cardiac output[2]. During late pregnancy, the enlarged uterus may obliterate flow in the caval vein leading to a gradual decrease of the elevated stroke volume.[2] Pulmonary arterial pressure and pulmonary vascular resistance decrease slightly. During pregnancy, mild degrees of valvular regurgitation are normal.

The overall effect of pregnancy is that the greater stroke volume increases the gradient over stenotic valve lesions, while the fall in systemic vascular resistance may decrease the grade of regurgitation.[2] Thus, regurgitant valve disease may actually improve during pregnancy, while stenotic valve disease may deteriorate. Patients with little or no symptoms are not at risk and generally have few problems. However, symptomatic patients often deteriorate. It is therefore advised to identify patients at risk before they become pregnant and treat them appropriately[2,4]. During labor, uterine contractions increase blood pressure and heart rate. Cardiac output and oxygen consumption therefore rise markedly. Cesarean section does not completely eliminate this effect and therefore is not necessarily tolerated any better in patients with symptomatic valve disease. However a primary Cesarean section is preferred above a secondary Cesarean section. After delivery, venous return immediately increases to compensate for blood loss. Heart rate, stroke volume and colloid-osmotic pressure decrease.[2, 4]

STENOTIC VALVE LESIONS

During pregnancy, mitral stenosis is more common than aortic valve stenosis. Pulmonary stenosis is mostly congenital, treated in childhood, and offers less problems during pregnancy.[2, 3] Tricuspid valve stenosis is rare.

In all cases of stenotic valve disease during pregnancy, treatment should be performed before conception.[2, 3] However, if significant valve disease is present during pregnancy, the amount of physical activity should be limited to prevent a high heart rate, dangerous changes in cardiac output, and potentially adverse effects on the fetal blood flow. Pharmacological treatment with ß-blockers results in an improvement of left ventricular filling and exercise tolerance, and has little adverse maternal or neonatal effects. Pregnancy increases the incidence of arrhythmias, particularly atrial fibrillation. If supraventricular arrhythmias occur, rate control with verapamil and ß-blockers is preferred above digoxine.

Every patient with atrial fibrillation needs anticoagulation with low molecular heparin[13,14], albeit a slight risk for mother and child. Occasionally it is necessary to relieve valve stenoses with balloon valvuloplasty, commissurotomy, valve repair of valve replacement.[2, 4]

Mitral Valve Stenosis

The incidence of rheumatic fever has decreased markedly in North America and Europe. However, women who migrated from countries where rheumatic fever is still endemic might still have had rheumatic fever in the past. Therefore, every obstetrician and cardiologist should be aware of the possibility of valvular pathology in these women. The natural history of mitral stenosis often shows a 20-25 year period without any symptoms. Therefore, the first symptoms might occur during pregnancy.

Patients with mitral valve stenosis typically complain of dyspnea, orthopnea and fatigue. Patients with a preexisting pulmonary hypertension may present with hemoptysis. Since this may be a life threatening complication –albeit rare- the prognosis is fairly bad [2,15].

Diagnosis of mitral stenosis by auscultation (a loud first heart sound and opening snap with diastolic rumble) may be difficult because of the location of the murmur under the enlarged left breast, and the physiological increase of the first heart sound during pregnancy. Diastolic murmurs during pregnancy, however, should always be evaluated by echocardiography. The presence of resting tachycardia, low pulse pressure, elevated jugular venous pressure, accentuated pulmonary components of the second heart sound, right ventricular lift, ascites and edema, should alarm the physician for possible presence of mitral stenosis[16]. Electrocardiography demonstrating left atrial enlargement and right axis deviation, with or without right ventricular hypertrophy, should do the same. Pregnancy induced increase of heart rate shortens left ventricular filling time. This increases left atrial pressure and decreases cardiac output (see also Table 1).[3] Pregnant women with mitral valve stenosis have a high risk of atrial fibrillation,[6] due to the high left atrial pressure and the intrinsic arrhythmologic effect of pregnancy. During atrial fibrillation there is no atrial contraction, which furthers impairs cardiac output. When the ventricular following rate is high, cardiac output it may rapidly decrease even further. Sometimes also the pulmonary artery pressure rises, which may lead to right ventricular failure in a small group of patients. Patients with advanced mitral stenosis have a high mortality risk during pregnancy (Table 1).[2, 3, 6, 13]

Treatment of mitral stenosis may include restriction of salt intake, while oral diuretic therapy may be considered. However, hypovolemia should be avoided since this increases heart rate, decreases filling pressures and thereby may lead to an insufficient cardiac output.[2, 13]

The delivery and post-partum period are most dangerous to women with mitral stenosis.[4, 6] During labor the further physiological increase in cardiac output and heart rate, may cause an even greater increase in left atrial pressure and decrease of filling time. These may lead to a fulminant pulmonary edema and cardiogenic shock.[2, 3] Post partum, the decrease in colloid-osmotic pressure and increase in venous return may further attribute to rapid development of pulmonary edema. Therefore, invasive monitoring with a Swan-Ganz catheter is advised, and the patient should sit upright when possible. Oxygen supply may lower the pulmonary pressure. Epidural anesthesia may be beneficial because it lowers pulmonary artery and left atrial pressures via peripheral vasodilatation. Endocarditis prophylaxis is not recommended. Generally, women with mitral stenosis may deliver vaginally. However, patients with severe hemodynamical problems may need a caesarian section. Current practice suggests that infants born from women with no or little symptoms of mitral stenosis have no significant perinatal mortality (Table 1).[2, 6, 7] With the interventions previously described, even neonates from women with severe mitral stenosis can be delivered with few complications.[6, 7] However, maternal mortality still occurs.[2, 6, 13]

Aortic Valve Stenosis
Congenital anomalies such as congenital bicuspid valves are more likely to compromise hemodynamics in pregnant women than rheumatic aortic valve stenosis (Table 1). However, severe aortic stenosis due to congenital disease is rare in the childbearing age. Most pregnant women with symptomatic aortic stenosis have been diagnosed in childhood, and the severity of their disease should be evaluated before conception.

Pregnant women complaining of dyspnea, chest pain and syncope, should be checked for aortic valve stenosis. Presyncope is common during normal pregnancy, but overt collapses are rare. The systolic murmur is more easily detectable because of its radiation over the carotids. These patients commonly develop a fourth heart sound that should always be regarded as abnormal. Again, in cases of doubt, echocardiography is advised.[5] Patients with a reduced left ventricular ejection fraction (<0.55) are at high risk for the development of heart failure. Patients with a gradient >50 mm Hg in early pregnancy should be followed by echo-doppler (Table 1).[5] Prophylactic aortic valve replacement[2, 3, 6] should be considered if the valve area is <1.0 cm^2. Pregnancy predisposes to aortic dissection by the hormonal effects on connective tissue, particularly patients with bicuspid aortic valves or Marfan's disease (see also *acute aortic valve regurgitation*). Acute chest pain should be a warning sign![2, 9-12]

Pregnant women with aortic stenosis are at risk of ventricular arrhythmias. Ambulatory ECG monitoring or implantable cardioverter-defibrillators should be considered.

Treatment depends on the symptoms and severity of stenosis. Patients with mild stenosis are unlikely to require intervention (table 1). Moderate stenosis can usually be managed medically with frequent follow-up. Severe stenosis should be considered for intervention with valvuloplasty or aortic valve replacement.[2, 3] A percutaneous approach is preferred if possible. Surgical intervention carries risk for the fetus. However, aortic valve replacement may be necessary in severely symptomatic patients with significant calcification or severe accompanying aortic insufficiency.[2, 3, 6]

During delivery, hemodynamic monitoring might not be necessary in most cases of aortic stenosis.[2, 3] However, in order to maintain sufficient pressure, pain control should be only given in low doses. Only patients with previous endocarditis, valvulotomy or prosthetic valves should be given antibiotic prophylaxis.[2]

The outcome of pregnancy in aortic stenosis seems to be fairly good.[7] Although there are few data on this matter, reports have been given of successful births with little complications in mother and child, even with severe stenosis.[2, 3, 7]

Pulmonary Valve Stenosis

Pulmonary valve stenosis is a congenital disease. Usually it is detected in early childhood by the auscultatory finding of a systolic ejection click and a murmur.[2]

Treatment of patients with a maximal gradient of >50 mm Hg, is performed by valvulotomy. Most women with pulmonary stenosis have been treated earlier or have little or no symptoms, and tolerate pregnancies well. Only patients with right ventricular failure or arrhythmias may be difficult to treat.[2, 3]

Any progression of symptoms as exercise intolerance, dyspnea and chest pain, should be closely surveyed.[6] The presence of an outflow murmur is inconclusive, as this can occur during normal pregnancy. However, echocardiography is indicated if the murmur progresses in duration and is accompanied by a prominent A-wave in the jugular venous pulse, right ventricular lift, systolic clicks and/or a systolic thrill over the pulmonic area.[5, 6] ECG's normally show right axis deviation and right ventricular hypertrophy.[2]

Treatment during pregnancy depends on symptoms. Symptomatic arrhythmias may occur, and should be treated depending on their origin. Percutaneous valvuloplasty is rarely necessary, but might be performed safely during pregnancy.[2]

Patients with little or no symptoms of their pulmonary stenosis during pregnancy, usually can safely deliver healthy babies.[2, 4, 6] Endocarditis prophylaxis is not required.[2]

Table 1. Maternal and/or Fetal Risk during Pregnancy in Valvular Pathology.

1.1 Type of valvular disease	1.2 High risk	1.3 Low risk
Mitral Valve Stenosis	Class II-IV	1. Class I-II, with LVEF >0.50 2. Mild to moderate, with MVA >1.5 cm^2, gradient <5 mmHg without severe pulmonary hypertension
Aortic Valve Stenosis	Severe with or without symptoms	Asymptomatic with mean gradient <50 mmHg and LVEF >0.50
Pulmonary Valve Stenosis	-	Mild to moderate
Mitral Valve Regurgitation	Class III-IV	Class I-II, with LVEF >0.50
Aortic Valve Regurgitation	1. Class III-IV 2. In Marfan syndrome	Class I-II, with LVEF >0.50
Pulmonary Hypertension in Aortic and/or Mitral pathology	Severe (>75% of systemic pressure)	Mild
Left Ventricular Dysfunction in Aortic and/or Mitral pathology	LVEF <0.40	LVEF >0.50
Prosthetic Valve	Mechanical Prostheses, requiring anticoagulation	Bioprosteses, not requiring anticoagulants

Adapted from Bonow et al.[3] Symptoms are qualified as NYHA functional classes; LVEF, left ventricular ejection fraction; MVA, mitral valve area.

REGURGITANT VALVE PATHOLOGY

Valve regurgitation normally gives no problems during pregnancy. Severe cases of regurgitation over any valve are rare in the childbearing age, and most patients are asymptomatic or present with relatively mild symptoms. Furthermore, the peripheral vasodilatation of pregnancy reduces the degree of regurgitation. In addition, the increase in heart rate reduces the diastolic interval, which may decrease the regurgitant volume in case of aortic regurgitation. Therefore, most women (even with severe degrees of regurgitation), tolerate their pregnancies well, often even improving in their symptoms.[2, 3] Most patients do not require any specific therapy. Occasionally it is advised to limit physical exercise and salt and fluid intake.

Prophylactic antibiotics are only advised for patients with earlier events of endocarditis. Patients with symptomatic arrhythmias may need treatment with ß-blockers. Invasive treatment is rarely required. Labor and delivery is generally safe and no specific therapy is needed normally. Most women with regurgitant disease deliver healthy children. Only neonates from mothers on ß-blockade should be checked for bradycardia or respiratory depression.[2]

Mitral Valve Regurgitation

A small degree of mitral insufficiency is common (up to 45% of women) in normal pregnancy. Most cases of pathological mitral regurgitation are caused by mitral valve prolapse. Rheumatic mitral regurgitation is becoming rare in the last ten years, and is often complicated by an associated mitral stenosis. Other –rare- causes are lupus erythematosus, the antiphospholipid antibody syndrome and the after-effects of infective endocarditis. Acute mitral regurgitation due to ruptured chordae tendinae or valve perforation due to bacterial endocarditis is very rare during pregnancy, but always very severe.[2]

Women with mitral regurgitation in the childbearing age, usually still have a well-functioning adaptive cardiac mechanism to volume overload. Their disease has rarely progressed to severe states. However, in few cases, the constant unloading of the left ventricle into the left atrium has already resulted in a reactive pulmonary hypertension, left ventricular enlargement and right-sided heart failure. The presence of cardiomegaly, atrial fibrillation and right-sided decompensation is associated with elevated maternal risks. In these patients, it might be necessary to reduce afterload by diuretics, nitrates or direct vasodilators, as long as hypotension is prevented. Nonetheless, generally even these women improve during pregnancy.[2]

Symptoms of mitral regurgitation are atypical and difficult to distinguish during pregnancy. Auscultatory finding of a midsystolic click and a systolic apical murmur radiating to the axilla should warn the physician. Most patients are diagnosed prior to pregnancy any way. However, diagnosis and evaluation is nearly always made by echocardiography. Careful examination of associated pathology (stenosis!) should be performed to assess risk factors.[3, 5] Notwithstanding the rarity of complications; incidents of infective endocarditis, thromboembolic events and sudden death have been reported in patients with severe mitral regurgitation.[2]

Aortic Valve Regurgitation
Chronic. Causes for aortic insufficiency are often bicuspid valves or aortic root disease. It induces left ventricular volume overload and dilatation. Generally, left ventricular function is well maintained until after the childbearing age. Pregnant women with exertional fatigue of NYHA class II or IV are rare, but they are at risk of progressive heart failure in the course of their pregnancy.[2, 3] Any progression of exertional fatigue must be considered an indication of decompensation. Syncope is often a sign of arrhythmias in ventricular dysfunction. Other symptoms of aortic regurgitation are aspecific and difficult to distinguish during pregnancy. However, systolic hypertension, wide pulse pressure and a blowing diastolic murmur should be a warning sign.[2]

Chronic aortic regurgitation, even severe, is often well tolerated in pregnancy. Symptoms may be treated with ß-blockers, diuretics and afterload reduction with direct vasodilators. However, hypotension should be prevented because it can cause placental hypoperfusion.

Labor and delivery is usually uncomplicated in patients with good left ventricular function. However, the rise in blood pressure during contractions can worsen the amount of regurgitation, and may be treated by vasodilators.

Acute (Aortic dissection). Patients with a bicuspid aortic valve or aortic root disease are at risk for acute aortic insufficiency due to proximal aortic dissection.[11] Approximately 50% of the dissections seen in women under 40 years of age occur during pregnancy.[9-12] It has been suggested that the hormonal changes of pregnancy in itself are responsible for weakening of the aortic tissue, but this has never been proven.[9,11,12]. Possibly the systemic hypertension, associated with many pregnancies, is responsible.[11] Nonetheless, even in pregnant patients with predisposing factors such as hypertension, Marfan's syndrome, bicuspid aortic valves or aortic root disease, acute dissection is very rare.[9-12]

When it occurs chances of survival for mother and child are very low.[9-12] Only when there is no rupture of the aortic wall, there are some chances of survival.[9] However, even if the patient initially survives, the proximal aortic dissection induces an acute aortic insufficiency.[2] The only other cause for acute aortic valve insufficiency is acute bacterial endocarditis (associated with intravenous drug abuse).[2]

Case reports have been published about successful treatment of mother and child by a combination of cesarean section and surgical intervention.[9-12] The order and urgency of both varies per author and per case report. One author suggests that medical treatment involving strict antihypertensive management is the preferred approach for type B aortic dissection.[12] Since this complication generally occurs during the third trimester or labor,[9, 11] the gestational age of the fetus often allows survival if the interventions were successful. Nonetheless, maternal and fetal mortality is very high. It has been suggested that patients with a high risk for dissection should have surgical repair during the first or second trimester of pregnancy and delivery by cesarean section.[9] Considering the rarity of this serious complication, the question remains whether this solution is sensible, since it induces an operative risk for mother and non-viable child.

PROSTHETIC HEART VALVES

Valve replacement during pregnancy should be avoided, if possible. This is currently feasible in most cases with intensive follow-up of obstetrician and cardiologist and adequate pharmacological treatment. There is little information available about the outcome of valve surgery during pregnancy. However, case reports suggest that it may be performed in the second trimester or at term after cesarean section.[2]

Pregnancy in women after valve replacement induces an increased resting gradient across the valve. This rarely causes difficulties in women with no or NYHA class I-II symptoms. It may be useful to perform a stress echocardiography in patients with NYHA class III-IV symptoms prior to conception. The response to an increase in cardiac output then can be registered. Women with left ventricular hypertrophy or small aortic roots after aortic valve replacement are at risk of developing high transvalvular gradients over the valve. Bioprostheses have a limited durability, particularly in the young patient with mitral valve disease. Pregnancy seems to accelerate the degenerative process further.[2, 8] Increased calcium turnover is blamed for this.[8] This may lead to urgent valve replacement during pregnancy and maternal death.[2, 8] Generally, bioprostheses are not used for younger patients.

An additional problem of pregnancy in women with prosthetic valves is the need for anticoagulation. The physiological chances of pregnancy include hyper-coagulability, thereby increasing the risk of thromboembolism. Patients with mechanical valves, prior thromboembolism, and/or atrial fibrillation require long-term anticoagulation.[2, 7, 8] However, data on anticoagulation during pregnancy are limited and conflicting. Antiplatelet agents have been shown to be ineffective during pregnancy.[8] Coumarin derivatives may cause an embryopathy when administered during the first trimester. It may also cause fetal hemorrhage, and increases the risk of life-threatening maternal hemorrhage during delivery.[2, 7] Nonetheless, some authors report successful coumarin treatment throughout pregnancy, and the number of embryopathies appears to be very low.[2, 7, 8] Other authors suggest that heparin treatment might be safer, possibly as a replacement for coumarin in the first and last trimester.[2, 7] However, thromboembolic events and retroplacental hemorrhage are much more common during heparin treatment.[2, 7, 8]

The outcome of pregnancy in patients with valve prostheses is generally good.[2, 7, 8] However, there is a higher chance for pre-term delivery and low weight babies.[7] It has been reported that women with bioprostheses do slightly better than those with mechanical valves (83% versus 73% healthy babies). The number of maternal death seems to be slightly higher in patients with mechanical valves,[8] possibly due to the fact that bioprostheses are less used in patients with severe cardiac pathology. There is little effect of anticoagulation on the outcome of pregnancy.[8]

DISCUSSION AND CONCLUSIONS

Valvular pathology is quite rare in pregnancy. However, it is may be a condition with considerable risks to mother and child and therefore should not be overlooked.

Female children with congenital valve disease and young women with rheumatic heart disease should be carefully be examined and counseled before conception. Early valve replacement might be considered. The prosthesis of choice, however, remains debatable. Mechanical prostheses carry the problem of anticoagulation, but have the advantage of durability. Bioprostheses often do not require anticoagulation but may deteriorate rapidly in young patients, particularly during pregnancy. However, the available literature on bioprostheses in young patients discusses allografts. The suggestion has been made that homografts might have greater durability. The problem remains that allografts are rarely available. In any fertile patient with identified valvular pathology, her physical condition should be optimized before pregnancy. Furthermore, it should be considered beforehand, which medical treatment might be necessary and available. In current practice, the outcome of pregnancy can be good. Nonetheless, it should be noted that the existing experience is limited, and studies upon this subject are based on retrospective data in small numbers of patients.

Pregnant women with unnoticed or untreated valvular pathology still may occur. The total number is small, and most patients have suffered rheumatic fever. However, since normally there is an asymptomatic period of 20-25 years and pregnancy amplifies symptoms, it is not exceptional when an expecting patient is diagnosed for the first time. In every patient with a history of rheumatic fever, migration from endemic countries or intravenous drug abuse, the possibility of valvular disease should be considered. Complaints of fatigue, dyspnea, orthopnea and malleolar edema before pregnancy should also warrant caution. Again, outcome of pregnancy can be good, but morbidity and mortality of mother and child still occurs in too many cases. The experience with rheumatic valvular pathology has been longer and in greater numbers than with valvular prostheses. Nonetheless, since rheumatic fever mostly causes stenotic valvular disease, the prognoses during pregnancy are certainly not better.

Mild degrees of regurgitant valvular disease are very common during pregnancy and have no consequences for therapy or outcome. Severe cases are very rare and normally documented from childhood. Optimization of the patient's condition before conception is, again, the strategy of choice. However, patients at risk for aortic dissection should be examined very carefully. If the risk is high and prenatal treatment is not possible, it might be advised to withdraw from reproduction.

REFERENCES

1. Rokey, R. Hsu, H.W., Moise, K.J., et al. (1994) Inaccurate noninvasive mitral valve area calculation during pregnancy, Obstet. Gynecol. 84, 950-955

2. Teerlink, J.R and Foster, E. (1998) Valvular heart disease in pregnancy, Cardiology clinics 16, 573-598

3. Bonow et al. (1998) ACC/AHA task force report. JACC 32, 1486-1582

4. Oakley, C.M. (1996) Valvular disease in pregnancy, Curr. Opin. Cardiol. 11, 155-159

5. Otto, C.M., Easterling, T.R., Benedetti, T.J. (1997) Role of echocardiography in the diagnosis and management of heart disease in pregnancy, in C.M. Otto (ed.): The practice of clinical echocardiography. W.B. Saunders Philadelphia, pp. 495-519

6. Siu, S.C., Sermer, M., Harrison, D.A., et al. (1997) Risk and predictors for pregnancy-related complications in women with heart disease, Circulation 96, 2789-2794

7. Caruso, A., De Carolis, S., Frazzani, S., et al (1994) Pregnancy outcome in women with cardiac valve prosthesis, Eur J. Ob. Gyn. & reproductive Biol.54, 7-11

8. Sbarouni, E. (1994) Outcome of pregnancy in women with valve prostheses, Br. Heart J.71, 196-201

9. Williams, G.M., Gott, V.L., Brawley, R.K., et al. (1988) Aortic disease associated with pregnancy, J. Vasc. Surg. 8, 470-475

10. Winkler, U., Edel, G., Fiedler, V., et al. (1987) Das aneurysma dissecans – eine seltene aber schwere komplication der schwangerschaft, Z. Geburtsh. U. Perinat. 191, 76-79

11. Pumphrey, C.W., Fay, T. and Weir, I. (1986) Aortic dissection during pregnancy, Br. Heart J. 55, 106-108

12. Zeebrechts, C.J., Schepens, M.A., Hameeteman, T.M., et al. (1997) Aortic dissection complicating pregnancy, Ann. Thorac. Surg. 64, 1345-1348

13. Wee Shian Chan, JG Ray. Low molecular weight heparin use during pregnancy: Issues of Safety and Practicality. Obstetrical and Gyneacology Survey 54, 1999: 649-654.

14. Gillis S, Shisnan A, Eldor A. Use of low molecular weight heparin for prophylaxis and treatment of thromboembolism in pregnancy. Int. J. Gynaecol. Obstet. 1992; 39: 297-301.

15. Narasimhan C., Joseph G., Thomas C.S.: Propanolol for pulmonary oedema in mitral stenosis.

16. Int. J.Cardiol. 44: 178-179, 1994.

17. Morley C.A., Lim B.A.: The risk of delay in diagnosis of breathlessness in pregnancy. B.M.J. 311:

18. 1083-1084, 1995.

SURGICAL APPROACH OF ACTIVE ENDOCARDITIS

A.H.M. VAN STRATEN

INTRODUCTION

Infective endocarditis (IE) of a native heart valve (NVE) or a prosthetic valve (PVE) may lead to fatal outcome for the patient. Antibiotic treatment will sometimes fail. Prompt or delayed surgical intervention may be indicated. According to recent literature the indication for operation, the principles of surgical technique and results of surgery in infective endocarditis are analyzed. Surgical techniques in aortic and mitral valve endocarditis will be discussed separately.

INDICATIONS FOR SURGICAL INTERVENTION

Persistent sepsis
Persistent sepsis for more than 72 hours is an indication for surgical intervention except when it is caused by streptococci. In terms of survival, septic patients do benefit more from surgical treatment than from medical treatment [1]. In IE caused by streptococci without clinical apparent complications, surgical intervention is indicated if fever exists beyond 10 days of adequate antibiotic treatment [2].

Type of infecting organism
In non-staphylococcal PVE in hemodynamically stable patients, medical therapy was as successful as surgical therapy[3]. In a group of patients with staphylococcal endocarditis, it was noted that the time between the initial fever and the occurrence of a trombo-embolic event was shorter than for patients with IE caused by another organisms[4]. Therefore, urgent surgical intervention should be considered in staphylococcal and fungal endocarditis [1,4,5,6].

Focal neurologic deficit
Compared to a group of patients suffering from IE and a focal neurologic deficit treated medically, a group of patients, treated with surgical intervention within 1 week of the neurologic event, did have a better outcome[7]. In a group of patients with staphylococcus endocarditis, who received medical therapy, mortality was significantly increased when the

central nervous system was involved[8]. Another study showed a significantly better survival in a group of patients operated within 72 hours after the initial cerebral embolism as compared with medical treatment [9].

Arterial embolisation
The risk of arterial embolisation appeared to decrease after 2 weeks of antibiotic treatment [10]. The benefit of surgery in avoiding embolic events will be the greatest in the early phase of IE. In one study it was noted that, when the vegetation size was more than 5 mm on ECHO, the cumulative freedom of thrombo-embolism was 45%. A first thrombo-embolism was follow in 54% by recurrent thrombo-embolism within 30 days [1]. In another study vegetations, sized larger than 1 cm, on the mitral valve, appeared to be associated with higher risk of embolisation[11]. Vegetations on the anterior leaflet of the mitral valve had the highest risk (37%) of embolisation [12]. Therefore, surgical intervention should be considered when large vegetations are detected on the mitral valve, particularly on the anterior leaflet and after the first major embolic event, when other complicating factors are present [13].

Annular abscess, ruptured aneurysm of the sinus and AV-block
Perivalvular abscesses are more common in PVE than in NVE, since the primary site of infection in PVE is the annulus. The weakest portion of the aortic annulus is near the membraneous septum and the atrio-ventricular node. This explains why a heart-block is a frequent sequela. Under the influence of systemic pressures abscesses may rupture or lead to fistulae. Only a small number of patients with annular abscess may be treated successfully with medical therapy [14].

Congestive heart failure (CHF)
CHF may develop acutely from perforation of a native or bioprosthetic-valve leaflet, ruptured chordae, valve obstruction from bulky vegetations, intra-cardiac shunts or dehiscence of a prosthetic valve. It may also develop more insidiously because of worsening of the valve incompetence and/or ventricular dysfunction. Time interval between the onset of cardiac failure and surgery was a significant risk factor for mortality [15]. In case of cardiac failure or impending cardiac failure, urgent surgical intervention is indicated since the prognosis is better with surgical intervention than with medical treatment [1,16].

Prosthetic valve dehiscent in PVE
For obvious reasons surgical intervention is indicated in case of prosthetic valve dehiscence.

Renal failure
One study showed that surgical intervention in case of renal failure had a better prognosis than medical treatment [1].

SURGICAL TECHNIQUE

Mitral valve endocarditis
The goal of all surgical interventions in infective valve endocarditis is to remove all infected tissue and to restore valve function. After removal of all infected tissue in mitral valve endocarditis, it is sometimes possible to preserve the native valve. Several techniques, that can be used to repair the defects in the native mitral valve, have been described [17]. A defect in one of the leaflets can be closed by a pericardial patch. Quadrangular resection of a part of the posterior leaflet together with ruptured chordae can be performed followed by repair of the leaflet. A triangular resection of the anterior leaflet can be done for the same reason. Another technique to resolve the problem of chordal rupture of the anterior leaflet is chordal transfer or chordal replacement with Gore-Tex sutures[18]. Annular dilatation can be resolved by implanting one of the available annuloplasty rings or by annuloplasty techniques without using a ring. If the destruction of the valve is more extensive the valve has to be replaced. Possible valve substitutes are mechanical prostheses, bioprostheses or homografts[19]. In extensive destruction of the valve and the annulus, the left atrium can become dehiscent from the left ventricle. Continuity must be restored. A pericardial patch or a Dacron patch can be used to restore the continuity of the left atrium and the left ventricle [20]. Abscess cavities can be filled with fibrin glue with or without antibiotic solution or with bio-degradable gentamycin swabs[21]. A prosthetic valve is implanted, fixed to the patch.

Aortic valve endocarditis
After resection of all infected tissue it is sometimes not possible to implant a mechanical valve or a bioprosthesis. In case of annular abscess or annular destruction or aortic root involvement sub-annular implantation of a homograft[22,23], a stentless porcine bioprosthesis[24] or a pulmonary autograft[25] may solve the problem. Other techniques are Teflon felt reconstruction [26], Dacron patch reconstruction [27] or insertion of a prosthetic heart valve in the ascending aorta with bypass grafts to the coronary arteries [28].

RESULTS OF SURGERY

Survival
In one study, risk factors for early and late mortality after surgical intervention in infective endocarditis appeared to be: increased age, preoperative neurologic complications, preoperative cardiogenic shock and mitral valve endocarditis[29]. I another study it was shown that, in addition to these risk factors, the presence of staphylococci and preoperative renal failure increased the rate of early mortality [30]. Another reported risk factor for increased early mortality was infection in multiple annuli in a patient group with annular abscesses [20]. However, in another study, the presence of only annular abscesses was reported not to be an independent risk factor [31]. In a patient group with perivalvular

abscesses, risk factors for survival were: older age, staphylococcal infection, fistulization and preoperative renal failure [32]. Other reported risk factors for early mortality were active infection at the time of surgery [5,33] and concomitant procedures [34]. In one study PVE was regarded as a risk factor in mitral valve PVE, whereas the activity of the infection was not a risk factor [35]. Reported operative mortality for "healed" endocarditis was 7% versus 14% in active endocarditis [5]. Reported operative mortality for PVE was 13-22% [5,30,36] and for NVE 6-7,5% [5,29,30].

Recurrent endocarditis
Activity of the infection appeared to be a risk factor for recurrent endocarditis. In aortic valve endocarditis the rate of recurrence of endocarditis is significantly higher in active endocarditis than with healed endocarditis [5,37]. Freedom from recurrent endocarditis after 5 years was 96% in the healed group and 89% in the active infected group[5]. In another study it was shown, that the risk of recurrent endocarditis after 8 years was 7% [29]. Presence of an annular abscess appeared to be a risk factor for recurrent endocarditis also [38].

Effect of type of valve substitute on survival and morbidity
Early mortality was the same with mechanical valves as with bioprostheses in retrospective studies[20,39]. The risk of recurrent endocarditis was higher with bioprostheses than with mechanical valves, 28% versus 8%, leading to more reoperations[39]. Early as well as late survival appeared to be better when a homograft was used instead of a prosthetic valve in a patient group with periannular abscess as reported in one retrospective study [40]. Reported rate of recurrence of endocarditis after implantation of a mechanical prosthesis was 2-8% [30,39,41], after implantation of a bioprosthesis 28% [39], after implantation of a homograft 2-3% [40,42] and after the Ross procedure 3% [25,43].

DISCUSSION

Traditional indications for early surgical intervention in active infective endocarditis are: congestive heart failure, persistent infection despite adequate antibiotics and recurrent arterial emboli. According to recent literature there are some additional indications. Infection with staphylococcus aureus or fungi in combination with other complicating factors is an indication for urgent operation. The risk of surgical intervention after focal neurologic deficit is less than the risk of medical treatment. Presence of vegetations larger than 1 cm on the anterior leaftlet of the mitral valve indicates urgent operation because of the high risk of embolisation. Regarding the several described surgical techniques and the different valve substitute, literature is not conclusive. No prospective randomized trials are available, answering the important question which valve substitute is superior. In general, it is better to avoid implanting prosthetic material in infected tissue. The radical resection of all infected tissue is probably more important than the type of implanted material. In mitral valve endocarditis, reconstructive surgery avoids the implantation of large amounts of prosthetic material. In aortic valve endocarditis, the pulmonary autograft has the advantage that vital tissue is used for implantation. However, the surgically demanding technique, which has to be performed in critically ill patients, seems to be a disadvantage. The advantage of homograft is the possibility to perform a subannular implantation in case of annular destruction, which avoids the implantation of Teflon, Dacron or pericardium patches.

REFERENCES

1. Horstkotte D, Schulte HD, Bircks W. Factors influencing prognosis and indication for surgical intervention in acute native-valve endocarditis. Infective Endocarditis by D Horstkotte and E Bodnar.

2. Kurland S, Enghoff E, Landelius J, Nystrrom SO, Hambraeus A, Friman G. A 10-year retrospective study of infective endocarditis at a university hospital with special regard to the timing of surgical evaluation in S. viridans endocarditis. Scan J Infect Dis 1999;31:87-91

3. Truninger K, Jost CH, Seifert B, Vogt PR, Follath F, Schaffner A, Jenni R. Long-term follow up of prosthetic valve endocarditis: what characteristics identify patients who were treated successfully with antibiotics alone? Heart 1999;82:714-20

4. Iemura J, Wakaki N, Saga T, Oka H, Oku H, Shirotani H. Timing of surgical treatment for native valve endocarditis. Jpn Circ J 1997;61:467-70

5. Aranki SF, Santini F, Adams DH, Rizzo RJ, Couper GS, Kinchla NM, Gildea JS, Collins JJ, Cohn LH. Aortic valve endocarditis. Determinants of early and late morbidity. Circulation 1994;90:II175-82

6. Rahal JJ, Simberkoff MS. Treatment of fungal endocarditis. In:Treatemnt of infective endocarditis. Bisno AL (ed), New York, Grune and Stratton 1981,pp 135-46

7. Parrino PE, Kron IL, Rross SD, Shockey KS, Kron AM, Towler MA, Tribble CG. Does a focal neurologic deficit contraindicate operation in a patient with endocarditis? Ann Thorac Surg 1999;67:59-64

8. Roder BL, Wnadall DA, Frimodt-Moller N, Espersen E, Skinhoy P, Rosdahl. Clinical features of staphylococcus aureus endocarditis: a 10 year experience in Denmark. Arch Intern Med 199´ 159:462-9

9. Horstkotte D, Piper C, Wiemer M, Arendt G, Steinmetz H, Bergemann R, Schulte HD, Schultheiss HP. Emergency heart valve replacement after acute cerebral embolism during florid endocarditis. Med Klin 1998;15:284-93

10. Steckelberg JM, Murphy JG, Ballard D, Bailey K, Tajik AJ, Taliercio CP, Giuliani ER, Wilson WR. Emboli in infective endocarditis: the prognostic value of echocardiography. Ann Intern Med 1991;114:635-640

11. Mugge A, Daniel WG, Frank G, Lichtlen PR. Echocardiography in infective endocarditis:reassessment of prognostic implications of vegetation size determined by the transthoracic and the transesophageal approach. J Am Cardiol J 1989;14:631-38

12. Rohrmann S, Erbel S, Gorge G, Makowski T, Mohr-Kahaly S, Nixdorff S, Drexler M, Meyer J. Clinical relevance of vegetation localisation by transesophageal echocardiography in infective endocarditis. Eur Heart J 1992;13:446-52

13. Bayer AS, Bbolger AF, Taubert KA, Wilson W, Steckelberg J, Karchmer AW, Levison M, Chambers HF, Dajani AS, Gewitz MH, Newsburger JW, Gerber MA, Shulman ST, Pallasch TJ, Gage TW, Ferrieri P. Diagnosis and management of infective endocarditis and its complications. Circulation 1998;98:2936-48.

14. Kunis RL, Sherrid MV, McCabe JB, Grieco MH, Dwyer EM jr. Successful medical therapy of mitral annular abscess complicating infective endocarditis. J Am Cardiol 1986;7:953-55

15. Colombo T, Lanfranchi M, Passini L. Quaini E, Russo C, Vitali E, Pellegrini A. Active infective endocarditis: surgical approach. Eur J Cardiothorac Surg 1994;8:15-24

16. Croft CH, Woodward W, Alliott A. Analysis of surgical versus medical therapy in active complicated native valve infective endocarditis. Am J Cardiol. 1983;51:1650

17. Carpentier A. Cardiac valve surgery – the "French correction". J Thorac Cardiovasc Surg 1983;86:323-37

18. David TE, Bos J, Rakowski H. Mitral valve repair by replacement of chordae tendineae with polytetrafluoroethylene sutures. J Thorac Cardiovasc Surg 1991;101:495-501

19. Gulbins H, Kreuzer E, Haushofer M, Uhlig A, Reichart B. Homografts for mitral valve replacement in florid endocarditis-an alternative to prosthetic replacement. Z Kardiol 1999;88:363-8

20. D'Udekem Y, David TE, Feindel CM, Armstrong S, Sun Z. Long-term results of operations for paravalvular abscess. Ann Thorac Surg 1996;62:48-53

21. Deyerling W, Haverich A, Potel J, Hetzer. A suspension of fibrin glue and antibiotic for local treatment of mycotic aneurysms in endocarditis- An experimental study. Thorac Cardiovasc Surgeon 1984;32:369-372

22. Glazier JJ, Verwilghen J, Donaldson RM, Ross DN. Treatment of complicated prosthetic aortic valve endocarditis with annular abscess formation by homograft aortic root replacement. J Am Coll Cardiol 1991;17:1177-82

23. Dossche KM, de la Riviere AB, Morshuis WJ, Schepens MA, Defauw JJ, Ernst SM. Cryopreserved aortic allografts for aortic root reconstruction: a single institution's experience. Ann Thorac Surg 1999;67:1617-22

24. Santini F, Musazzi A, Bertolini P, Pugliese P, Fabbri A, Faggian G, Prioli A, Mazzucco A. Stentless porcine bioprostheses in the treatment of aortic valve infective endocarditis. J Card Surg 1995;10:205-9

25. Niwaya K, Knott-Craig CJ, Santangelo K, Lane MM, Chandrasekaran K, Elkins RC. Advantage of autograft and homograft valve replacement for complex aortic valve endocarditis. Ann Thorac Surg 1999;67:1603-8

26. Ergin MA, Raissi S, Follis F, Lansman SL, Griepp RB. Annular destruction in acute bacterial endocarditis. Surgical techniques to meet the challenge. J Thorac Cardiovasc Surg 1989;97:755-63

27. Bailey WW, Ivey TD, Miller DW. Dacron patch closure of aortic annulus mycotic aneurysms. Circulation 1982;66:SI-126-130

28. Danielson GK, Titus JL, Dushane JW. Successful treatment of aortic valve endocarditis and aortic root abscesses by insertion of prosthetic valve in ascending aorta and placement of bypass grafts to coronary arteries. J Thorac Cardiovasc Surg 1974;67:443-97

29. Jault F, Gandjbakhch I, Rama A, Nectoux M, Bors V, Vaissier E, Nataf P, Pavie A, Cabrol C. Active native valve endocarditis: Determinants of operative death and late mortality. Ann Thorac Surg 1997;63:1737-41

30. Bauernschmidt R, Jacob HG, Vahl CF, Lange R, Hagl S. Operation for infective endocarditis: Results after implantation of mechanical valves. Ann Thorac Surg 1998;65:359-64

31. Danchin N, Retournay G, Stchepinski O, Selton-Suty C, Voiriot P, Hoen B, Canton P, Villemot JP, Mathieu P, Cherrier F. Comparison of long-term outcome in patients with or without aortic ring abscess treated surgically for aortic valve infective endocarditis. Heart 1999;81:177-81

32. Choussat R, Thomas D, Isnard R, Michel PL, Iung B, Hanania G, Mathieu P, David M, du Roy de Chaumaray T, De Gevigney G, Le Breton H, Logeais Y, Pierre-Justin E, de Riberolles C, Morvan Y, Bischoff N. Perivalvular abscesses associated with endocarditis: clinical features and prognostic factors of overall survival in a series of 233 cases. Perivalvular abscesses French multicentre Study. Eur Heart J;1999:20:232-41

33. Ladowski JS, Deschner WP. Allograft replacement of the aortic valve for active endocarditis. J Cardiovasc Surg (Torino) 1996;37:S61-2

34. Petrou M, Wong K, Albertucci M, Becker SJ, Yacoub MH. Evaluation of unstented aortic homografts for the treatment of prosthetic aortic valve endocarditis. Circulation 1994;)0:II198-204

35. Aranski SF, Adams DH, Rizzo RJ, Couper GS, Sullivan TE, Collins JJ, Cohn LH. Determinants of early mortality and late survival in mitral valve endocarditis. Circulation 1995;92(9 suppl):II143-9

36. Lyttle BW. Surgical treatment of prosthetic valve endocarditis. Semin Thorac cardiovasc Surg 1995;7:13-9

37. Grover FL, Cohen DJ, Oprian C, Henderson WG, Sethi G, Hammermeister KE. Determinants of the occurence of and survival from prosthetic valve endocarditis. Experience of the veterans affairs cooperative study on valvular heart disease J Thorac Cardiovasc Surg 1994;108:207-14

38. Pompilio G, Brockmann C, Bruneau M, Buche M, Amrani M, Louagie Y, Eucher P, Rubay J, Jamart J, Dion R, Schoevaerdts JC. Long-term survival after aortic valve replacement for native active infective endocarditis. Cardiovasc Surg 1998;6:126-32

39. Wos S. Jasinski M, Bachowski R, Piekarski M, cerglarek W, Domaradzki W, Gemel M, Wenzel-Jasinska I, Kadziola Z. Results of mechanical prosthetic replacement in active valvular endocarditis. J Cardiovas Surg (Torino) 1996;37(suppl):29-32

40. Knossalla C, Weng Y, Yankah AC, Siniawski H, Hofmeister J, Hammerschmidt R, Loebe M, Hetzer R. Surgical treatment of active infective aortic valve endocarditis with associated periannular abscess- 11 year results. Eur Heart J 2000;21:490-7

41. Gaudino M, De Filippo C, Pennestri F, Possati G. The use of mechanical prostheses in native aortic valve endocarditis. J Heart Valve Dis 1997;6:79-83

42. Dossche K, Brutel de la Riviere A, Morshuis W, Schepens M, Ernst J. Aortic root replacement with human tissue valves in aortic valve endocarditis. Eur J Cardiovasc Surg 1997;12:47-55

43. Petterson G, Tingleff J, Joyce FS. Treatment of aortic valve endocarditis with the Ross operation. Eur J Cardiothorac Surg 1998;13:678-84.

INDEX

Active endocarditis. *See* Endocarditis
Aneurysm of sinus, ruptured, with
    endocarditis, 192
Annular abscess, with endocarditis, 192
Annulus of mitral valve, size, perioperative
    transesophageal echocardiography,
    29–30
Aortic endocarditis, surgical technique,
    193–198
Aortic insufficiency
    aortic regurgitation, etiology of, 70
    aortic root ratio, 70
    aortic valve leaflets, 70
    bicuspid valve lesion, 72
    echocardiography, 70
    follow-up, 70
    imaging of, 95–96
    left ventricular hypertrophy, postoperative
        regression, 126
    Marfan's syndrome, 70, 72
    noninvasive follow up, 72
    outcome, factors influencing, 73–74
    preoperative evaluation, 69–76
    severity assessment, 70–71
        color flow evaluation, 70, 71
        in diastole, 71
        Doppler, 70
        exercise testing, 71
        grading, 71
        holodiastolic flow reversal, 71
        systole, 71
        two-dimensional echocardiographic
            examination, 70
    timing of surgical intervention
        for asymptomatic patients, 73
        for symptomatic patients, 72–73
Aortic leaflets, in aortic insufficiency, 70
Aortic prosthesis, patient mismatch,
    142–143, 143–147, 150
Aortic regurgitation
    decision to not operate, 157
    etiology of, 70
    in pregnancy, 185–186
Aortic root ratio, in aortic insufficiency, 70
Aortic stenosis

    decision to not operate, 155–156
    hemodynamic evaluation of, 77–84
        stenosis severity, 78–79
        low-flow states, 79–80
        valve morphology, 78
    imaging of, 94–95
    left ventricular hypertrophy, postoperative
        regression, 125–126
    in pregnancy, 182
Aortic valve replacement, mechanical
    prosthesis, 117–124
    autografts, 119
    availability, 120
    bioprostheses, 118, 119
    bleeding, 118
    comfort of patient, 121
    death, valve-related, 120
    hemodynamic performance, 118
    hemolysis, 119
    homografts, 119
    implantation technique, 121
    mechanical valves, 118
    periprosthetic leak, 119
    prosthetic valve endocarditis, 119
    reoperation, freedom from, 120
    stentless, 119
    structural valve failure, 119
    thrombo-embolism, 118
    valve thrombosis, 118
    valve-related morbidity, 118–120
Arterial embolisation, with endocarditis, 192
Artifacts, mechanical valves prone to, 100
Atrial fibrillation
    after mitral valve replacement, 46
    magnetic resonance imaging and, 94
Atrioventricular block, with endocarditis,
    192
Autografts, tissue valves, 106
Automatic implantable cardioverters,
    magnetic resonance imaging and, 94

Back flow in prosthetic valves, normal
    patterns, 39
Bicuspid valve lesion, 72

Bjork Shiley prosthetic valve, patient
    mismatch, 138, 139, 140, 141
Bleeding
    after mitral valve replacement, 48
    with mechanical prosthesis for aortic
        valve replacement, 118

Cardiac catherization, preoperative, mitral
    valve stenosis, 7
Cardioverters, magnetic resonance imaging
    and, 94
Carpentier Edwards prosthetic valve, patient
    mismatch, 138, 139, 140, 141
Chordal elongation, perioperative
    transesophageal echocardiography, 30
Claustrophobia, magnetic resonance
    imaging in patient with, 94
Cochlear implants, magnetic resonance
    imaging and, 94
Comorbidity, influencing decision to not
    operate, 159
Congestive heart failure, with endocarditis,
    192
Contraindications to magnetic resonance
    imaging, 94
Coronary angiography, mitral regurgitation,
    17

Decision not to operate, 155–162
    aortic regurgitation, 157
    aortic stenosis, 155–156
    comorbidity, influencing decision, 159
    mitral regurgitation, 157–158
    mitral stenosis, 158–159
Degenerative mitral valve, 32
Dehiscence
    prosthetic valve, with endocarditis, 192
    suture, after mitral valve repair, 37
Diastole, length of, magnetic resonance
    imaging and, 94

Echocardiography, 59–68
    after mitral valve surgery, 59–68
    aortic insufficiency, 70
    aortic valve, 85–87
    checklist for postoperative evaluation, 68
    goals of, 59–60
    intraoperative echo, use of, 59
    left ventricular function, 62–63
    mitral regurgitation, 17–18
        left ventricular function in, 62–63
        aortic dissection, 63
        right-sided problems, 63

mitral valve, 5–7, 18, 26–28, 30–32,
    35–37, 60–61, 61–62, 87–88
postoperative, 59–68
systolic anterior motion, mitral valve,
    predisposing factors, 68
transesophageal, 18
    anatomical structures, mitral view, 26
    annulus of mitral valve, size, 29–30
    aortic valve disease, 85–87
        postoperative evaluation, 87
        preoperative evaluation, 85–86
    back flow in prosthetic valves, normal
        patterns, 39
    chordal elongation, 30
    complications after mitral valve repair,
        37
        impaired left ventricular function, 37
        mitral stenosis, 37
        suture dehiscence, 37
    degenerative mitral valve, 32
    echocardiographer's view, mitral valve,
        26–28
    endocarditis mitral valve, 32
    four-chamber view, mitral valve, 26
    function of mitral valve, 28–30
    ischemia detection, 88–89
    ischemic mitral valve, 32
    long-axis view, mitral valve, 27
    mid-esophageal views, mitral valve, 26
    mitral regurgitation, 18
        mechanism of, 30–32
    mitral valve anatomy, 26
    mitral valve disease, 87–88
        postoperative evaluation, 88
        preoperative evaluation, 87–88
        proximal isovelocity surface area
            measurement, 87
        regurgitant jet area measurement, 87
    during mitral valve repair, 35–37
        late results, 36–37
        pitfalls, 36
    mitral-commissural view, mitral valve,
        27
    motion of mitral valve leaflets, 29
        excessive leaflet motion, 29
        normal leaflet motion, 29
        restricted leaflet motion, 29
    multiplane transesophageal
        echocardiography, 26
    perioperative, 27–44, 85–92
    position of mitral valve leaflets after
        closing, 28
        malapposition of leaflets, 29

malcoaptation of leaflets, 28
preload measurement, 89
prosthesis evaluation, transesophageal
    echocardiography, 38–41
  anatomic abnormality assessment, 38
  prosthetic valve leakage, 39–41
  prosthetic valve obstruction, 38–39
rheumatic mitral valve, 32
segmental wall-motion scoring system,
    89
severity, mitral regurgitation, 33–35
  jet area assessment, 33
  method selection, 35
  proximal convergence zone,
      assessment of size, 34
  proximal jet diameter, 33
  pulmonary venous flow, assessment
      of, 34–35
  severity, mitral regurgitation,
      surgical assessment, 35
systolic function, 89
transesophageal echocardiography,
    mechanism of mitral regurgitation,
    30–32
transgastric basal short-axis view,
    mitral valve, 27
transgastric basal two-chamber view,
    mitral valve, 27
transgastric mid short-axis view, mitral
    valve, 27
transgastric views, mitral valve, 26
two-chamber view, mitral valve, 27
Electrocardiogram, preoperative, mitral
    valve stenosis, 4
Electronical devices, magnetic resonance
    imaging and, 94
Embolisation, arterial, with endocarditis, 192
Endocarditis
  annular abscess, 192
  arterial embolisation, 192
  atrioventricular block, 192
  congestive heart failure, 192
  focal neurologic deficit, 191–192
  indications for, 191–192
  mitral valve, 32
  mitral valve replacement, 49, 52
  prosthetic valve, 119
    dehiscence, 192
  renal failure, 192
  results of surgery, 193–194
    recurrent endocarditis, 194
    survival, 193–194
    type of valve substitute, 194

ruptured aneurysm of sinus, 192
  sepsis, persistent, 191
  surery, 191–198
  surgery, technique, 193
    aortic valve endocarditis, 193
    mitral valve endocarditis, 193
  type of infecting organism, 191
Exercise hemodynamics, cardiac
    catheterisation with, mitral
    regurgitation, 17

Flow rate calculation, PISA method, mitral
    regurgitation, 19
Four-chamber view, mitral valve, 26
Function of mitral valve, 28–30

Hemodynamic evaluation of aortic stenosis,
    77–84
  stenosis severity, 78–79
  low-flow states, 79–80
  valve morphology, 78
Hemodynamic measurements, magnetic
    resonance imaging, 94
Hemorrhage, after mitral valve replacement,
    52
Holodiastolic flow reversal, in aortic
    insufficiency, 71
Hrombosis, with mechanical prosthesis for
    aortic valve replacement, 118
Hypertension, after mitral valve
    replacement, 49–50
Hypertrophy, left ventricular, postoperative
    regression, 125–136
  aortic insufficiency, 126
  aortic stenosis, 125–126
  left ventricular remodeling, 127–130
  mitral insufficiency, 131–132

Imaging techniques, 93–104. *See also under*
    specific imaging technique
  aortic valve insufficiency, 95–96
  aortic valve stenosis, 94–95
  artifacts, mechanical valves prone to, 100
  atrial fibrillation, degrades image quality,
    94
  claustrophobia, 94
  cochlear implants, 94
  diastole, variable length of, 94
  electronical devices, 94
  magnetic resonance imaging
    contraindications to, 94
    technical aspects, 93–94

mechanical valves, in magnetic resonance environment, 100
mitral valve regurgitation, 97–98
mitral valve stenosis, 96–97
mixed valvular disease, 99–100
pacemakers, 94
prosthetic valves, 100
pulmonic valve disease, 99
Starr-Edwards valve, in magnetic resonance environment, 100
tricuspid valve disease, 99
International Ross Registry, 113. *See also* Ross procedure
Intraoperative echocardiography, 59
during mitral valve repair, 35–37
late results, 36–37
pitfalls, 36
Ischemia detection in peri-operative period, transesophageal echocardiography, 88–89
Ischemic mitral valve, 32
Isovelocity surface area measurement, mitral valve disease, 87

Leak, periprosthetic, with mechanical prosthesis for aortic valve replacement, 119
Left ventricular function
after mitral valve repair, 37
intraoperative echocardiography, 62–63
Left ventricular hypertrophy, postoperative regression, 125–136
aortic insufficiency, 126
aortic stenosis, 125–126
left ventricular remodeling, 127–130
mitral insufficiency, 131–132
Left ventricular remodeling, postoperative regression, concomitant coronary artery disease with, 130
Long-axis view, mitral valve, 27

Magnetic resonance imaging
contraindications to, 94
technical aspects, 93–94
Marfan's syndrome, 70, 72
Mechanical prosthesis. *See also under* specific type of prosthesis
actuarial survival, 52
anatomic abnormality assessment, 38
aortic valve replacement, 117–124
atrial fibrillation, 46
availability, 120
bioprostheses, 118, 119

bleeding, 48, 52, 118
comfort of patient, 121
complications, 52
death, valve-related, 120
endocarditis, 49, 52, 119, 192
evaluation, transesophageal echocardiography, 38–41
hemodynamic performance, 118
hemolysis, 119
homografts, 119
imaging of, 100
implantation technique, 121
late survival after
postoperative determinants for, 47
pre-operative determinants for, 46
leakage, 39–41
left ventricular failure, 52
in magnetic resonance environment, 100
mechanical valves, 118
mitral incompetence, natural history of, 46
mitral valve, 45–58
obstruction, 38–39
paravalvular defects, 51, 52
patient mismatch, 137–154
periprosthetic leak, 119
in pregnancy, 186–187
prosthetic valve endocarditis, 119
pulmonary hypertension, post-operative, 49–50
reoperation, 48–49, 52, 120
freedom from, 120
right ventricular failure, 52
stentless, 119
structural deterioration, 52
structural failure, 50, 119
structural valve failure, 119
sudden death, 52
thromboembolism, 48, 52, 118
valve dysfunction, 163–178
non-structural dysfunction, 168–169, 177–178
orientation, 163–165, 173–176
structural dysfunction, 166–168
subvalvular apparatus, 165–166
valve orifice area, patient mismatch, 137–138
indexed for body surface area, 137
valve thrombosis, 51, 52, 118
valve-related morbidity, 118–120
Medtronic Freestyle prosthetic valve, patient mismatch, 139
Medtronic Hall prosthetic valve, patient mismatch, 138, 139, 140, 141

Midesophageal views of mitral valve, 26
Mismatch, between valve prosthesis, patient,
    137–154
  aortic valve prosthesis, 142–143, 150
  assessment, 137–143
  Bjork Shiley prosthetic valve, 138, 139,
      140, 141
  Carpentier Edwards prosthetic valve, 138,
      139, 140, 141
  clinical impact, 143–147
    aortic valve prosthesis, patient
        mismatch, 143–147
    mitral valve prosthesis, patient
        mismatch, 148–150
  Medtronic Freestyle prosthetic valve, 139
  Medtronic Hall prosthetic valve, 138, 139,
      140, 141
  mitral valve prosthesis, 143, 150
  prosthetic valve orifice area, 137–138
    indexed for body surface area, 137
  St. Jude prosthetic valve, 138, 139, 140,
      141
  Starr Edwards prosthetic valve, 138, 139,
      140, 141
Mitral regurgitation
  age, influence on timing of surgery, 21
  angiography, cardiac catheterisation with,
      17
  calculation of, regurgitant orifice area, 19
  cardiac index, influence on timing of
      surgery, 21
  cause of mitral regurgitation, evaluation
      of, 16–17
  contractile dysfunction, detecting onset
      of, 20
  coronary angiography, 17
  coronary artery disease, presence of,
      influence on timing of surgery, 21
  decision to not operate, 157–158
  echocardiography, 17–18
  exercise hemodynamics, cardiac
      catheterisation with, 17
  flow rate calculation, PISA method, 19
  functional class, influence on timing of
      surgery, 21
  hemodynamic variables, influence on
      timing of surgery, 21
  imaging of, 97–98
  infectious endocarditis, 16
  ischemic mitral regurgitation, 17
  jet area assessment, 33
  left atrial dilation, 16

  left ventricular dilation, systolic
      dysfunction, 17
  left ventricular function in, 19–20, 62–63
    aortic dissection, 63
    right-sided problems, 63
  mean pulmonary artery pressure,
      influence on timing of surgery, 21
  method selection, 35
  mitral annular calcification, 16
  mitral leaflets, chordae, impairment of, 16
  mitral valve closure, 16
  non-invasive imaging, 17
  in pregnancy, 184–185
  preoperative evaluation, 15–24
  proximal convergence zone, assessment
      of size, 34
  proximal jet diameter, 33
  pulmonary venous flow, assessment of,
      34–35
  regurgitant fraction, transvalvular driving
      pressure and, 19
  right heart catheterisation, 17
  severity evaluation, 17–19, 33–35
    grading, 18
    underestimation of, 18
  signal attenuation, apical views, 18
  surgical assessment, 35
  systolic dysfunction, left ventricle, 21
  timing of surgery, 20
    factors influencing, 21
  transesophageal echocardiography, 18
  transvalvular driving pressure, color flow
      indices, 19
  valve leaflets, 17
  ventriculography, 17
Mitral stenosis
  after mitral valve repair, 37
  asymptomatic, evaluation algorithm, 10
  balloon angioplasty, 8
  cardiac catherization, 7
  chest x-ray, 4
  decision to not operate, 158–159
  diagnostic testing, 4
  echocardiography, 5–7, 8
  electrocardiogram, 4
  evaluation algorithm, 11, 12
  history, 3
  imaging of, 96–97
  physical examination, 4
  in pregnancy, 181–182
  preoperative evaluation, 3–14
  treatment guidelines, 9–12
    asymptomatic patients, 9–10

class II symptoms, 10–11
class III-IV symptoms, 11–12
valvulotomy, suitability for, 7–9
Mitral valve anatomy, 26
Mitral valve disease, 87–88. *See also under*
specific disease
proximal isovelocity surface area
measurement, 87
regurgitant jet area measurement, 87
Mitral valve endocarditis, surgical
technique, 193–198
Mitral valve function, 28–30
Mitral valve prosthesis, patient mismatch,
143, 148–150, 150
Mitral valve repair, postoperative
evaluation, 60–61
Mitral valve replacement, postoperative
evaluation, 61–62
Mixed valvular disease, imaging of, 99–100
Motion of mitral valve leaflets, perioperative
transesophageal echocardiography, 29
excessive leaflet motion, 29
normal leaflet motion, 29
restricted leaflet motion, 29
Multiplane transesophageal
echocardiography, 26

Not operating, decision regarding, 155–162
aortic regurgitation, 157
aortic stenosis, 155–156
comorbidity, influencing decision, 159
mitral regurgitation, 157–158
mitral stenosis, 158–159

Orifice area, prosthetic valve, patient
mismatch, 137–138
indexed for body surface area, 137

Pacemakers, magnetic resonance imaging
and, 94
Pannus, mitral valve replacement and, 51–52
Perioperative transesophageal
echocardiography, 27–44, 85–92
aortic valve disease, 85–87
postoperative evaluation, 87
preoperative evaluation, 85–86
echocardiographer's view, mitral valve,
26–28
function of mitral valve, 28–30
intraoperative transesophageal
echocardiography during mitral
valve repair, 35–37
late results, 36–37

pitfalls, 36
ischemia detection, 88–89
mitral valve disease, 87–88
postoperative evaluation, 88
preoperative evaluation, 87–88
proximal isovelocity surface area
measurement, 87
regurgitant jet area measurement, 87
multiplane transesophageal
echocardiography, 26
preload measurement, 89
segmental wall-motion scoring system, 89
systolic function, 89
Periprosthetic leak, with mechanical
prosthesis for aortic valve replacement,
119
Physiological adaptation, in pregnancy, 180
PISA method, flow rate calculation, mitral
regurgitation, 19
Porcine xenografts, tissue valves, 105–106
Position of mitral valve leaflets after closing,
perioperative transesophageal
echocardiography, 28
malapposition of leaflets, 29
malcoaptation of leaflets, 28
Postoperative echocardiography after mitral
valve surgery, 59–68
checklist for postoperative evaluation, 68
goals of, 59–60
intraoperative echo, use of, 59
left ventricular function, 62–63
mitral regurgitation, left ventricular
function in, 62–63
aortic dissection, 63
right-sided problems, 63
mitral valve repair, postoperative
evaluation, 60–61
mitral valve replacement, postoperative
evaluation, 61–62
systolic anterior motion, mitral valve,
predisposing factors, 68
Postoperative regression
left ventricular hypertrophy, 125–136
aortic insufficiency, 126
aortic stenosis, 125–126
left ventricular remodeling, 127–130
mitral insufficiency, 131–132
left ventricular remodeling, concomitant
coronary artery disease with, 130
Pregnancy, valvular pathology in, 179–190
physiological adaptation, 180
prosthetic heart valves, 186–187
regurgitant valve pathology, 184–186

aortic valve regurgitation, 185–186
  mitral valve regurgitation, 184–185
stenotic valve lesions, 180–184
  aortic valve stenosis, 182
  mitral valve stenosis, 181–182
  pulmonary valve stenosis, 183
Preoperative evaluation of aortic
    insufficiency, 69–76
  aortic regurgitation, etiology of, 70
  aortic root ratio, 70
  aortic valve leaflets, 70
  bicuspid valve lesion, 72
  echocardiography, 70
  follow-up, 70
  Marfan's syndrome, 70, 72
  noninvasive follow up, 72
  outcome, factors influencing, 73–74
  severity assessment, 70–71
    color flow evaluation, 70, 71
    in diastole, 71
    Doppler, 70
    exercise testing, 71
    grading, 71
    holodiastolic flow reversal, 71
    systole, 71
    two-dimensional echocardiographic
        examination, 70
  timing of surgical intervention
    for asymptomatic patients, 73
    for symptomatic patients, 72–73
Preoperative evaluation of mitral
    regurgitation, 15–24
  age, influence on timing of surgery, 21
  angiography, cardiac catheterisation with,
      17
  calculation of, regurgitant orifice area, 19
  cardiac index, influence on timing of
      surgery, 21
  cause of mitral regurgitation, evaluation
      of, 16–17
  contractile dysfunction, detecting onset
      of, 20
  coronary angiography, 17
  coronary artery disease, presence of,
      influence on timing of surgery, 21
  echocardiography, 17–18
  exercise hemodynamics, cardiac
      catheterisation with, 17
  flow rate calculation, PISA method, 19
  functional class, influence on timing of
      surgery, 21
  hemodynamic variables, influence on
      timing of surgery, 21

infectious endocarditis, 16
ischemic mitral regurgitation, 17
left atrial dilation, 16
left ventricular dilation, systolic
    dysfunction, 17
left ventricular function, 19–20
mean pulmonary artery pressure,
    influence on timing of surgery, 21
mitral annular calcification, 16
mitral leaflets, chordae, impairment of, 16
mitral valve closure, 16
mitral valve repair, 16
noninvasive imaging, 17
regurgitant fraction, transvalvular driving
    pressure and, 19
regurgitant severity, underestimation of,
    18
right heart catheterisation, 17
severity, evaluation of, 17–19
signal attenuation, apical views, 18
systolic dysfunction, left ventricle, 21
timing of surgery, 20
    factors influencing, 21
transesophageal echocardiography, 18
transvalvular driving pressure, color flow
    indices, 19
valve leaflets, 17
ventriculography, 17
Preoperative evaluation of mitral valve
    stenosis, 3–14
  asymptomatic mitral stenosis, evaluation
      algorithm, 10
  balloon angioplasty, 8
  cardiac catherization, 7
  chest x-ray, 4
  diagnostic testing, 4
  echocardiography, 5–7, 8
  electrocardiogram, 4
  evaluation algorithm, 11, 12
  history, 3
  physical examination, 4
  treatment guidelines, 9–12
    asymptomatic patients, 9–10
    class II symptoms, 10–11
    class III-IV symptoms, 11–12
  valvulotomy, suitability for, 7–9
Prosthesis. *See also under* specific type of
    prosthesis
  actuarial survival, 52
  anatomic abnormality assessment, 38
  aortic valve replacement, 117–124
  atrial fibrillation, 46
  autografts, 119

availability, 120
bioprostheses, 118, 119
bleeding, 48, 52, 118
comfort of patient, 121
complications, 52
death, valve-related, 120
endocarditis, 49, 52, 119, 192
evaluation, transesophageal
    echocardiography, 38–41
hemodynamic performance, 118
hemolysis, 119
homografts, 119
imaging of, 100
implantation technique, 121
late survival after
    postoperative determinants for, 47
    pre-operative determinants for, 46
leakage, 39–41
left ventricular failure, 52
mechanical valves, 118
mitral incompetence, natural history of, 46
mitral valve, 45–58
obstruction, 38–39
pannus, 51–52
paravalvular defects, 51, 52
patient mismatch, 137–154
periprosthetic leak, 119
in pregnancy, 186–187
prosthetic valve endocarditis, 119
pulmonary hypertension, post-operative,
    49–50
reoperation, 48–49, 52, 120
right ventricular failure, 52
stentless, 119
structural deterioration, 52
structural failure, 50, 119
sudden death, 52
thromboembolism, 48, 52, 118
valve dysfunction, 163–178
    non-structural dysfunction, 168–169,
        177–178
    orientation, 163–165, 173–176
    structural dysfunction, 166–168
    subvalvular apparatus, 165–166
valve orifice area, patient mismatch,
    137–138
    indexed for body surface area, 137
valve thrombosis, 51, 52, 118
valve-related morbidity, 118–120
Pulmonary hypertension, after mitral valve
    replacement, 49–50
Pulmonary valve stenosis, in pregnancy, 183
Pulmonic valve disease, imaging of, 99

Recurrent endocarditis, 194
Regurgitant jet area measurement, mitral
    valve disease, 87
Regurgitation
    aortic
        decision to not operate, 157
        etiology of, 70
        in pregnancy, 185–186
    mitral
        age, influence on timing of surgery, 21
        angiography, cardiac catheterisation
            with, 17
        annular calcification, 16
        calculation of, regurgitant orifice area,
            19
        cardiac index, influence on timing of
            surgery, 21
        cause of mitral regurgitation, evaluation
            of, 16–17
        closure, 16
        contractile dysfunction, detecting onset
            of, 20
        coronary angiography, 17
        coronary artery disease, presence of,
            influence on timing of surgery, 21
        decision to not operate, 157–158
        echocardiography, 17–18
        exercise hemodynamics, cardiac
            catheterisation with, 17
        flow rate calculation, PISA method, 19
        functional class, influence on timing of
            surgery, 21
        hemodynamic variables, influence on
            timing of surgery, 21
        imaging of, 97–98
        infectious endocarditis, 16
        ischemic mitral regurgitation, 17
        jet area assessment, 33
        leaflets, chordae, impairment of, 16
        left atrial dilation, 16
        left ventricular dilation, systolic
            dysfunction, 17
        left ventricular function, 19–20, 62–63
            aortic dissection, 63
            right-sided problems, 63
        mean pulmonary artery pressure,
            influence on timing of surgery, 21
        method selection, 35
        non-invasive imaging, 17
        in pregnancy, 184–185
        preoperative evaluation, 15–24

proximal convergence zone, assessment of size, 34
proximal jet diameter, 33
pulmonary venous flow, assessment of, 34–35
regurgitant fraction, transvalvular driving pressure and, 19
regurgitant severity, underestimation of, 18
right heart catheterisation, 17
severity evaluation, 17–19, 33–35
signal attenuation, apical views, 18
surgical assessment, 35
systolic dysfunction, left ventricle, 21
timing of surgery, 20
    factors influencing, 21
transesophageal echocardiography, 18
transvalvular driving pressure, color flow indices, 19
valve leaflets, 17
valve repair, 16
ventriculography, 17
in pregnancy, 184–186
aortic valve, 185–186
mitral valve, 184–185
Renal failure, with endocarditis, 192
Rheumatic mitral valve, 32
Right heart catheterisation, mitral regurgitation, 17
Ross, Donald, 111. See also Ross procedure
Ross procedure in aortic valve disease, 111–116
advantages of, 112
disadvantages of, 113
International Ross Registry, 113
results of, 113–114
Ruptured aneurysm of sinus, with endocarditis, 192

Segmental wall-motion scoring system, 89
St. Jude prosthetic valve, patient mismatch, 138, 139, 140, 141
Starr Edwards prosthetic valve
in magnetic resonance environment, 100
patient mismatch, 138, 139, 140, 141
Stenosis. See also under type of stenosis
decision to not operate with, 155–156
Stentless mechanical prosthesis, for aortic valve replacement, 119
Structural prosthetic valve dysfunction, 166–168
Subvalvular apparatus, prosthetic valve dysfunction, 165–166

Surgical procedures
endocarditis, active, 191–198
hemodynamic evaluation, of aortic stenosis, 77–84
imaging techniques, 3–44, 59–76, 93–104. See also under specific imaging technique
left ventricular hypertrophy, postoperative regression of, 125–136
perioperative transesophageal echocardiography, 27–44
postoperative evaluation, mitral valve surgery, 59–68
pregnancy, 179–190
preoperative evaluation
aortic insufficiency, 69–76
mitral regurgitation, 15–24
mitral valve stenosis, 3–14
prosthesis
for aortic valve replacement, 117–124
for mitral valve replacement, 45–58
patient mismatch, 137–154
Ross procedure, 111–116
timing of, 15–24, 69–76, 155–162
tissue valves, 105–110
transesophageal echocardiography, in peri-operative period, 85–92
valve prosthesis, dysfunction of, 163–178
Suture dehiscence, after mitral valve repair, 37
Systolic anterior motion, mitral valve, predisposing factors, 68

TEE. See Transesophageal echocardiography
Thromboembolism
after aortic valve replacement, 118
after mitral valve replacement, 48, 52
Timing of surgical procedures, 15–24, 69–76, 155–162. See also under specific procedure
Tissue valves, 105–110
autografts, 106
indications for use of, 108
porcine xenografts, 105–106
Transesophageal echocardiography, 18
anatomical structures, mitral view, 26
annulus of mitral valve, size, 29–30
aortic valve disease, 85–87
postoperative evaluation, 87
preoperative evaluation, 85–86
back flow in prosthetic valves, normal patterns, 39
chordal elongation, 30

complications after mitral valve repair, 37
  impaired left ventricular function, 37
  mitral stenosis, 37
  suture dehiscence, 37
degenerative mitral valve, 32
echocardiographer's view, mitral valve, 26–28
endocarditis mitral valve, 32
four-chamber view, mitral valve, 26
function of mitral valve, 28–30
ischemia detection, 88–89
ischemic mitral valve, 32
long-axis view, mitral valve, 27
mid-esophageal views, mitral valve, 26
mitral regurgitation, 18
  mechanism of, 30–32
mitral valve anatomy, 26
mitral valve disease, 87–88
  postoperative evaluation, 88
  preoperative evaluation, 87–88
  proximal isovelocity surface area measurement, 87
  regurgitant jet area measurement, 87
during mitral valve repair, 35–37
  late results, 36–37
  pitfalls, 36
mitral-commissural view, mitral valve, 27
motion of mitral valve leaflets, 29
  excessive leaflet motion, 29
  normal leaflet motion, 29
  restricted leaflet motion, 29
multiplane transesophageal echocardiography, 26
perioperative, 27–44, 85–92
position of mitral valve leaflets after closing, 28
  malapposition of leaflets, 29
  malcoaptation of leaflets, 28
preload measurement, 89
prosthesis evaluation, transesophageal echocardiography, 38–41
  anatomic abnormality assessment, 38
  prosthetic valve leakage, 39–41
  prosthetic valve obstruction, 38–39
rheumatic mitral valve, 32
segmental wall-motion scoring system, 89
severity, mitral regurgitation, 33–35
  jet area assessment, 33
  method selection, 35
  proximal convergence zone, assessment of size, 34
  proximal jet diameter, 33

pulmonary venous flow, assessment of, 34–35
severity, mitral regurgitation, surgical assessment, 35
systolic function, 89
transesophageal echocardiography, mechanism of mitral regurgitation, 30–32
transgastric basal short-axis view, mitral valve, 27
transgastric basal two-chamber view, mitral valve, 27
transgastric mid short-axis view, mitral valve, 27
transgastric views, mitral valve, 26
two-chamber view, mitral valve, 27
Transvalvular driving pressure, color flow indices, mitral regurgitation, 19
Tricuspid valve disease, imaging of, 99
Two-chamber view of mitral valve, 27

Valve prosthesis. See also under specific type of prosthesis
actuarial survival with, 52
anatomic abnormality assessment, 38
aortic valve replacement, 117–124
atrial fibrillation, 46
autografts, 119
bioprostheses, 118, 119
bleeding, 48, 52, 118
comfort of patient, 121
complications, 52
death, valve-related, 120
dysfunction, 163–178
endocarditis, 49, 52, 192
  with mechanical prosthesis for aortic valve replacement, 119
evaluation, transesophageal echocardiography, 38–41
hemodynamic performance, 118
hemolysis, 119
homografts, 119
imaging of, 100
implantation technique, 121
late survival after
  postoperative determinants for, 47
  pre-operative determinants for, 46
leakage, 39–41
left ventricular failure, 52
mechanical valves, 118
mitral incompetence, natural history of, 46
mitral valve, 45–58
morbidity, 118–120

non-structural dysfunction, 168–169, 177–178
obstruction, 38–39
orientation, 163–165, 173–176
pannus, 51–52
paravalvular defects, 51, 52
patient mismatch, 137–154
periprosthetic leak, 119
in pregnancy, 186–187
prosthetic valve endocarditis, 119
pulmonary hypertension, post-operative, 49–50
reoperation, 48–49, 52, 120
right ventricular failure, 52
stentless, 119
structural deterioration, 52
structural dysfunction, 166–168
structural failure, 50, 119
structural valve failure, 119
subvalvular apparatus, 165–166
sudden death, 52
thromboembolism, 48, 52, 118
thrombosis, 51, 52, 118
tissue, 105–110
   autografts, 106
   porcine xenografts, 105–106
valve orifice area, patient mismatch, 137–138
   indexed for body surface area, 137
valve thrombosis, 118
valve-related morbidity, 118–120
Valve surgery

endocarditis, active, 191–198
hemodynamic evaluation, of aortic stenosis, 77–84
imaging techniques, 3–44, 59–76, 93–104. *See also under* specific technique
left ventricular hypertrophy, postoperative regression of, 125–136
perioperative transesophageal echocardiography, 27–44
postoperative evaluation, mitral valve surgery, 59–68
pregnancy, 179–190
preoperative evaluation
   aortic insufficiency, 69–76
   mitral regurgitation, 15–24
   mitral valve stenosis, 3–14
prosthesis
   for aortic valve replacement, 117–124
   for mitral valve replacement, 45–58
   patient mismatch, 137–154
Ross procedure, 111–116
timing of, 15–24, 69–76, 155–162
tissue valves, 105–110
transesophageal echocardiography, in peri-operative period, 85–92
valve prosthesis, dysfunction of, 163–178
Valvulotomy suitability, with mitral valve stenosis, 7–9
Ventriculography, mitral regurgitation, 17

Xenografts, porcine, tissue valves, 105–106